How to Grow Your Own Herbs

A Guide to Growing and Cooking Herbs from Your Own Garden

Jake Ragen

Table of Contents

Introduction

Did you know that approximately 200 billion pounds of herbs and spices are produced each year by the United States of America alone? ("Herb and Spice History", 2023). Close to 55% of all households in the US have gardens, making it one of the top three gardening countries in the world. That number is only increasing each day, and an estimated 18 million people (Gardening Statistics (2024), 2024) in the US have started gardening in 2021. Everyone is doing their part in protecting the environment. You can too but start an herb garden.

Before we get into the details of herbs and herbal gardening, though, let's start at the very beginning.

What is an herb? There are many ways you can define herbs; a dictionary works best if you are looking for the scientific definition. But to keep things simple, we define herbs as any plant that contains seeds, flowers, and leaves that you can add to food to enhance its flavor or nutritional value. Any garden where you grow herbs is an herb garden, and you are an herbal gardener! You can use many herbs from your garden to create flavorful dinners.

Spices and herbs are not just used to enhance the flavor of your food, though. Many have medicinal properties as well. Chamomile—we all know this as a refreshing kind of tea—can help with anxiety and stress ("A Guide to Common Medicinal Herbs," n.d.). Thyme is another herb that contains important compounds that help treat bacterial infections and relieve coughing ("Thyme: Uses, Side Effects, and More," n.d.).

The best part about herbs like these—or any other herb as a matter of fact—is that they are so simple to grow and thrive in all kinds of environments, including urban gardens or other small spaces. Even if it seems like you have no space at all for a garden at home, herbs are small and "space-friendly" plants that can grow anywhere, like on a kitchen countertop, if there's some sunlight coming in.

"Urban Gardening" is a phrase that you might have come across on social media and it is becoming increasingly popular. It's a way of growing vegetables, fruits, and herbs in your own in small spaces, like balconies, patios, and windowsills, in urban areas. If you choose to grow herbs as part of your urban garden, that will make you an "herbal gardener." Growing your own food and herbs is not as difficult as it sounds. In fact, it's fun, relaxing, and easy! You might have seen many social media posts and interviews from avid gardeners talking about how relaxed they feel while tending to their gardens.

Spending time in the garden can be therapeutic and have so many health benefits. Have you noticed how your mood seems to be much better in the spring than in the winter? Just a few minutes of exposure to soil and sun can improve your mental and physical health. Gardening is also a sustainable practice that helps maintain biodiversity and combat climate change.

You might be thinking about how a small garden can help support such a large concept of biodiversity, right? The answer to that question is right here! Have you noticed how the temperature in urban areas is slightly higher than in rural areas? The reason for this is less greenery. When you manage an urban garden, you are creating a green space in the city— something that cities don't have a lot of. Heat gets trapped up in cities quickly, but trees, grass, and other plants can help slightly cool the area, which in turn minimizes the need for artificial cooling. This means that, by being an urban gardener, you are indirectly playing your part in keeping your city healthy and combating pollution. Keeping your hometown or city healthy is a collective task; urban gardening is you playing your role as part of that task.

Also, as an extra advantage, gardening counts as exercise! All the work you put in to grow plants—the trimming, watering, and maintenance— all of it will help burn a few calories. Plus, it's fresh food grown in a healthy way! All that pollution from growing, harvesting, storing, and transporting allows so many bacteria to enter your food and herbs. By growing them at home, you can avoid food that was subjected to these elements.

Growing your own herbs, like mint, thyme, rosemary, and others, can save you a lot of money. Rather than buying those plastic-wrapped herbs from the store, every time you want to use a bit, you can just go to your garden and pluck as much as you need. The plant stays fresh, so you spend almost nothing apart from a one-time investment!

Herbal gardening has numerous health benefits as well. For starters, you know what food is going into the plant you are growing, so you can be sure it's free from pesticides, chemical fertilizers, or other harmful chemicals.

When you grow your own food and herbs especially, you tend to try new flavor profiles. For example, if you have never tasted rosemary or thyme before, growing one of these plants might make you interested in finding ways to incorporate them into your dish. It also encourages you to eat healthier, home-cooked meals rather than ordering in or getting takeout. You might even get some inspiration from watching different videos on how people use these herbs in different cuisines across the world! The next time you're craving some Chinese or Indian food, you'll have all the herbs you need to make it at home waiting for you in your kitchen, literally!

It sounds exciting, doesn't it? Throughout this book, you will find ideas on how to start your herbal garden, how to grow different herbs, and finally harvest them when they are ready. You also get an understanding of what you can do with the herbs once they are grown.

Don't worry if you don't have a green thumb, though. Herbal gardening is for everyone! There are a lot of herbs that even a total beginner can grow and maintain perfectly well. You can also do this as a family activity with your kids to help them understand gardening and its importance at a young age. Anyone can be a gardener!

Chapter 1:

Horticulture for Beginners—The

Ins and Outs of Herbal Gardening

The thought of maintaining a garden seems like a tedious task at first, it's work all the way from buying products to sowing seeds, maintaining, and finally harvesting. Once you get started though, gardening is fun!

Our early ancestors, in all parts of the world, began gardening about 25,000 years ago (The Brief History of Container Gardening, n.d.). They grew their own food on nearby lands and fields, and spent time understanding how plants grow, what seasons they grow in, and how to make them survive harsh weather. Medicinal herbs were around for long before people knew how to write or record anything, and it's not just us humans who use these herbs. Studies show that animals like monkeys have been using herbs ("Monkeys and Medicinal Plants," 2011) to treat one of their biggest problems: parasites.

Since the weather in urban areas isn't as suitable for large-scale crops as it is in rural areas, we need to do some work around plant maintenance. City gardening is done on a much smaller scale, of course, but plants still need the same care and love. Gardeners in these urban areas find ways to help their plants withstand all kinds of weather and pollution by adapting to certain special technologies. If they can maintain a healthy garden, you can do it too!

This chapter will explain the basics of herb gardening and its benefits and uses.

Benefits of Herb Gardens

The basic and most obvious reason for you to have an herb garden is that it saves you money, and you will always have fresh herbs ready for you whenever you need them. On the days you cook, you might go to the store and spend a few dollars on herbs like mint, thyme, rosemary, etc. Once you use a little bit for the meal you are making, you have no idea what to do with the rest, right? You might just put them in the fridge, and they turn brown and unusable, or they just aren't as fresh the next time you need them. When that happens, you throw them away, and go to the store to buy them again, and the cycle continues.

With a garden, though, the herbs are always fresh and sitting right in front of you for you to pluck and use however much you need. As a bonus, they make the entire area smell so fresh!

Aside from just saving money, herb gardens have lots of other benefits. Dinner never gets boring. There's always a new flavor you can add to your food aside from the medicinal value they provide.

Herbs for Health

For centuries, herbs have been used for treating a wide variety of ailments, both simple and complex. Including these herbs as a part of your diet can prevent and even cure some illnesses. While at-home medication and herbs can help to a certain extent, it's important to keep in mind, however, that consultation with a doctor is necessary for any major health issue.

Though sometimes classified as a root vegetable or spice, garlic is an herb that a lot of people use every day in various cuisines around the world. Did you know that garlic is not just tasty, but also plays an important role in keeping your heart healthy? Studies ("Garlic for treating hypercholesterolemia: A meta-analysis of randomized clinical trials," 2000) show that garlic can help reduce cholesterol levels as well.

Ginger is another herb with high medicinal value. Studies show (Ginger for nausea and vomiting of pregnancy, 2016) that ginger can help reduce symptoms of nausea and vomiting and is especially beneficial for pregnant women.

Peppermint is another extremely popular herb that is known to treat headaches and aid digestion. Parsley has antioxidant properties and can help lower blood pressure. In a similar way, other herbs too have health benefits and having these plants at home can help boost the overall vitamin value of your meal.

Herbs for Flavor

Each herb is unique and has a special flavor that can make any dish taste so much better and make it healthier. The table below gives a description of some types of herbs, their flavors, and some ideas for using them.

Herb	Flavor	Ideas of Dishes
Mint	strong peppery flavor	drinks, salads
Oregano	earthy	sauces
Cilantro	fresh	used widely in Indian and Mexican cuisines.
Thyme	light lemon	soups, sauces, steak
Rosemary	pine	pork, lamb stews
Chives	light onion	can be used as a garnish in almost any dish
Basil	sweet, slightly spicy	pasta sauce, soup

The use of herbs does not need to be limited to the dishes listed in the table above, though. Each cuisine has a specific use for each herb and a unique way of imparting its flavor into the dish.

Gardening for Physical Activity

Just like a brisk walk or a light jog can burn a few calories, gardening can too. Gardening works out the most basic muscles in your body—thighs, arms, buttocks, back, and abdomen. Studies show (Gardening as Exercise, 2017) that by just watering your plants, you can burn about 60 calories a day. Weeding and trimming shrubs using manual tools can burn up to 180 calories—that is about as many calories as you would burn in 1.5 miles of jogging!

Enjoy a nice spring day in your garden with all your plants. If you have a lot of herbs, there's a soothing fragrance all around you! Be sure to take things slow on hot summer days and keep yourself hydrated if you are outdoors for more than 30 minutes.

Uses for Herbs

We have seen earlier on in this book that herbs have a wide variety of uses, both for flavor, and as medicine. Let us now take a look at some of these properties in detail.

Aesthetics

Maintaining a beautiful-looking garden while keeping in mind important factors like sunlight can seem like a tedious task. Lucky for you, though, herbs make this a little easier. They don't need large areas to grow or specific placement directions. Some varieties of herbs can survive on as little as two hours of sunlight and heat each day!

Most herbs even grow well next to each other in the same garden bed or container. Mint, however, is one type—and probably the only type—of herb that needs to be placed in its own pot, since it tends to 'take over' all the space it can.

Each herb has a different color and texture. Use this to your advantage. Make arrangements in different patterns based on the herb's shape, size, and color. Here are some ideas for growing an aesthetically beautiful herb garden.

Vertical Garden

Even if you don't have a lot of space in your garden or kitchen for plants, there is always enough space for herbs! The walls are a perfect place you can utilize to your advantage. Start by choosing the right wall. You need the wall to be able to support some weight, a few containers, soil, and plants. Next, select your materials to create a supportive structure on your wall—a vertical garden trellis—and make sure it is attached securely.

Next, add some soil to the pots and sow your seeds. Arrange your plants any way you want across the structure, and make sure you want them every day. In a few weeks, you should see your plants start to grow, and most herbs should be ready to harvest within a month.

If you have the option, you can even hang some pots that have handles from a curtain rod near your window.

Tabletop Garden

If you have an old table lying around in your home that you don't use anymore, you can always turn it into a garden table. Place it in a sunny corner inside or outside your house and start growing your plants. Make sure you put a plastic sheet or cardboard underneath your plants if you have them indoors, so the excess water that drains from the pot does not ruin your floors.

Here are a few ideas for containers

- teapot

- old blender jar

- used paint can

- water jug

- plastic storage containers

- milk cans

- mason jars

Anything can be a pot! You read that right—just about anything with small holes at the bottom can be used as a pot! It doesn't just have to go on the table, the kitchen counter, or close to the sink; it works perfectly!

Do you have a plastic serving bowl or a watering can that you no longer use? You can make some small holes at the bottom, give it a nice coat of paint on the outside, and turn it into a plant pot! Get creative with the painting. The design options are endless. You can even make the pot match the decor inside your house to give it an attractive look.

Bookshelf in the Balcony

Bookshelves are great ways to use vertical space and add layers of plants in a smaller space. Since these herb plants are generally small, you can fit quite a few pots on each layer and even use the top rack to add your favorite decorative elements. Some people like to add a small water fountain or a Buddha in their garden to represent peace.

You can also use pallets to create the same kinds of layers if you are on a budget. Pallets offer the same benefits, allowing you to create a series of layers and go as high as you want to.

Another idea is to arrange some pots on various sections of a ladder. This looks aesthetically pleasing and serves the purpose, which is the primary goal of decorating gardens. All of these ways make your garden look beautiful and help you stay organized. Organizing your garden using unique items like ladders is also a great conversation starter!

For vertical gardens, there are special watering systems that you can install to automatically water your plants and keep them fresh.

Herbs for Aromatherapy

Herbs don't necessarily need to be eaten. They can be used in aromatherapy as well. Aromatherapy is an alternative medicine that involves using essential oils to improve your physical and mental well-being. You can choose to inhale these oils through a diffuser—soak some leaves in water and light a candle underneath the diffuser. When the water evaporates, your room will smell fresh and start to show its effects.

Alternatively, you can go to a licensed therapist who can give you a massage for a set amount of time, incorporating these essential oils.

Inhaling these fragrances can help stimulate your nervous system and help your brain release serotonin and endorphins. Studies (Fung T.K. et al., 2021) show that these oils can have a positive effect on your mood. Aromatherapy is also sometimes used to treat menstrual cramps and help with pre-labor pains.

Like we've seen before, your home herb garden does not need to be confined to a particular area or space. Lavender, for example, has therapeutic effects that can trigger sleep and promote relaxation. Growing this plant in your bedroom can keep the area fragrant while allowing you to sleep better.

Garden sage is another example of an herb that can be used in aromatherapy to help you think better and cure headaches (Hadimpour M. et al., 2014). It has a slight floral and spicy fragrance, and can make your home smell relaxing.

Lemon balm, another herb with a pleasant lemon aroma, is proven to improve sleep quality (Loft A. et. al. 2020).

Culinary Uses of Herbs

There is no doubt that every single restaurant, however big or small, uses herbs in one way or another. Both dried and fresh herbs are used in dishes around the world to add flavor. Typically, most chefs use herbs towards the end of the cooking process to ensure the herb retains its flavor in the dish. Plants have endless potential, and when used correctly, they can elevate any simple dish. Using herbs can make a plain sauce, for example, much richer and more enjoyable.

Instead of ordering food when you feel like eating something flavorful, having an herb garden can inspire you to try and cook that same meal at home. Cooking can be a family activity. Even your kids can have some fun taking care of these plants and helping you harvest them.

The next time you think about ordering Mediterranean, Indian, Italian, or any other flavorful food, know that you can make the same meal at home in a much healthier and more delicious way by using homegrown plants. It's no lie that a home cooked meal tastes better and even brings about a special connection in your family.

Lotions and Creams

The world is always changing; herbal products are the trend now, and anything organic is beneficial over chemical products. Herbal oils, creams, lotions, and balms have been used for centuries. Ayurveda is a very old Indian concept that makes use of herbs to treat various ailments. Using the same concept, even today, various botanicals and herbs are used as lotions to treat skin irritation, pimples, acne, and other skin-related problems.

Store bought lotions and creams, especially organic ones, can get quite expensive. When you grow your own herbs, you can make these at home too. The advantage of putting in the effort is that you know what's going into them.

Here is a simple way for you—even as a total beginner—to be able to make your own homemade lotion. Its fragrance can be a great conversation starter!

Homemade Herbal Lotion

For this process, you will need a double boiler. If you don't have one, it's okay. You can make your own by placing a saucepan on the stove on high heat and filling it with water. Place another heat-resistant bowl on top of this to melt any ingredients you want. Fun fact: This is how you melt chocolate!

Ingredients for the lotion:

- one cup of distilled water

- ¾ cup of a carrier oil; this can be almond oil or coconut oil.

- half ounce of beeswax

- two or three drops of any essential oil of your choice (optional)

Steps to make it:

1. Whisk the oil and beeswax gently into a double boiler and keep whisking until your beeswax melts.

2. Allow this to cool completely, and then transfer it to a blender jar. You will notice that it's slightly thicker than it was when it was hot.

3. Turn the blender on high, and slowly add in the distilled water. Keep doing this until you see the mixture turn white and thicken. Be sure not to add in all the water at once; sometimes the mixture thickens after using just a half cup of water.

4. Stop blending once it's thick. If you are using herbal essential oils, add in a few drops at this point and slightly blend them.

5. Transfer this to an air-tight container.

This cream stays fresh for about a month in the fridge. It's also important to remember that if at any point during the blending process, your blender starts to get hot, stop blending and allow the mixture to cool down. The heat can spoil the texture and affect its shelf life.

Homemade Herbal Oil

Herbal oils are also very simple to make. Doing a simple massage with them can help relieve stress and muscle tension. Here are the steps and ingredients to make your own herbal oil.

Ingredients:

- 1 cup fresh herbs; you can use any herb of your choice depending on your need.

- ¾ cup carrier oil: cold-pressed oils like olive or almond work more effectively and are also body-safe.

- a teaspoon of salt

- water

- ice bath

Steps:

1. Pour some water into a saucepan and add salt. Allow the water to boil.

2. Add the herbs to this boiling water and let them blanch until they turn bright green. This usually takes under a minute.

3. Transfer the herbs into an ice bath and let them cool down completely.

4. Once cool, pat the herbs dry on a towel. Get as much moisture out as you can.

5. Transfer this to a blender and add in the oil.

6. Blend on high speed until everything is well combined.

7. Sieve this with a cheesecloth and transfer this into the mason jar.

This oil lasts fresh for about a week in the fridge and can be used for massages.

Medicinal Purposes of Herbs

The following table provides a better understanding of the medicinal properties of each type of herb.

Herb	Medicinal Use
Chamomile Flower	reduces inflammation and swelling
Ginger root	eases nausea
Feverfew Leaf	treats fever and help with migraine
Garlic	protects your heart
Basil	regulates blood sugar and lowers cholesterol
Evening Primrose	helps with PMS, and reduces symptoms of arthritis
Rosemary	antioxidant, anti-microbial
Thyme	helps fight acne, lowers heart rate, and improves immunity
Sage	anti-oxidant, lowers blood sugar
Mint	antibacterial, and can reduce stress
Parsley	reduces bloating

Teas Made with Herbs

Herbal teas taste truly amazing. Start your morning with a fresh, hot cup of herbal tea to elevate your mood and brighten your day. Here is a list of a few kinds of herbal teas you should try.

- chamomile tea

- peppermint tea

- hibiscus tea

- ginger tea

- lemon balm tea

Teas are so simple to make and have lots of nutrients that you need each day. Teas are medicine for the mind, body, and soul. You need to dehydrate your herbs carefully before you can make tea with them. There are quite a few ways to do this, including using a food dehydrator, oven, or even a microwave. In some countries—and even a few states in the US—herbs dry perfectly under the summer sun.

To dehydrate your herbs in the oven, spread each leaf of your herb onto a clean oven tray or baking sheet. Then, put them in the oven. Keep checking on them until they turn crispy like a leaf in the fall. This takes less than five minutes at that heat, so always be alert.

If you live in a place where it gets hot in the summer, you can dry your herbs outside. Spread your herbs onto a baking tray or a dinner plate and put them in a nice sunny spot outside. Make sure there isn't too much wind though, it can send them flying all over the place! In a few hours, your herbs should be crisp, dry, and ready.

There are a few more things you need to know when drying your fresh herbs. More information on drying and ways of storing them will be discussed in the later chapters.

Carefully crush the dried herbs and store them in an airtight container in a cool and dry place. Dried herbs have a very long shelf life; some can even last up to two years when stored properly.

Once your process of drying and storing is done, you are ready to make a fresh herbal tea every day!

1. Take a cup of water in a saucepan and turn the heat up to high.

2. Once the water is warm, add in a spoonful of your dried herbs and turn the heat down to low.

3. Allow this to boil and keep stirring occasionally.

4. Once it reaches a boil, take a tea strainer, and filter out your tea into a cup.

If you like the flavor, you can drink this directly or mix it in with half a spoon of honey. Honey is a better sweetener than sugar for teas because of its antioxidant properties.

Preparing for an Herbal Garden

Now that you know all about herbs, why to grow them, and how beneficial they are, it is time to learn about how exactly you can begin a garden and the practical steps involved in it.

If you have a backyard, it can be the perfect place for an herb garden. You can use a variety of large containers or even garden beds in the soil. Each herb can have its own space, and you don't really need to worry about them not getting enough sunlight. If you don't have a backyard, though, a kitchen windowsill works just as perfectly! There is always plenty of room indoors to grow all varieties of herbs.

First, identify what herbs you intend to grow and the amount of sunlight they need. Most herbs don't need to be placed in areas that get a lot of sunlight, but make sure the area you choose for your plants gets at least a little sunlight each day. Planning is the first step to making a garden work, so it is worth spending time making a drawing of your space, plant arrangements, and listing out the sunlight and water requirements of each plant. This will help you when you start potting, seeding, and decorating your garden.

Understanding your soil is another important factor in how your herbs will grow. Typical garden soil can be used for any kind of herbal plant. Ensure that there are proper holes for drainage at the bottom of your container; holes allow the excess water to drain from the plant and prevent the roots from rotting in the wet soil. For healthy growth, you can also mix your garden soil with some compost to make the soil richer and more fertile. Having a water source close to your plants, like a hose in a garden, is important to ensure your plants are able to get the water they need to grow healthy. For an indoor garden, a watering can would be enough for you to manually water potted plants.

There is no strict rule as to what herbs you should grow and shouldn't. You can grow as many varieties as you like, if you are willing to put in the effort to maintain them. If it's just for food and flavor, for example, you can grow about four or five varieties that you use, and that would be perfectly okay. If you are looking to transform your physical and mental health through aromatherapy and herbal teas, it is worth having a large garden with a wide variety of herbs in it.

Chapter 2:

Using Your Green Thumb—Caring

for Your Garden

Once you have a proper plan in mind for your garden, the next step is doing the actual planting. Whether you are starting from a seed or buying a grown plant, it's important to maintain the plant and provide it with ample sunlight and water so it grows and stays healthy.

Selecting the Right Soil

At any regular gardening store, there are quite a few different types of soil. You know that soil is the foundation of a garden, but how do you know which soil is the right choice to pick?

For most herbs and vegetables, you need to pick a soil that has a good blend of silt, clay, sand, and contains organic matter. All these are important to provide the nutrients your plant needs to grow and lead a healthy life. A soil that is very dark in color and crumbles when you touch it is a sign of being good quality.

If you can't find soil that suits your specific needs or if you are unsure about the soil you just bought, you can nourish it by creating homemade compost. Compost is easy to make, but the entire process is slow. You need to start making your compost at least a month or two before spring to ensure that it is ready in time.

Enrich Your Soil with Compost

To make compost, start by collecting your green and brown material. Green material includes kitchen scraps and anything that is uncooked, like vegetable peels. Fill a medium-sized basket with it. You can add to this basket every day or after each meal. Next, collect your brown material, such as paper scraps, dried leaves and twigs, or garden waste. You will need more brown material than green, so plan accordingly.

Chop up your green material into small pieces. Smaller pieces decompose easily, which will speed up the composting process. Do the same with your brown material. Break the twigs into small pieces and rip paper into tiny bits.

Next, take a big plastic bucket and poke some holes at the bottom to allow drainage. Alternatively, you can find compost buckets online or at gardening centers, that are designed for this exact purpose. Start creating layers of green and brown, adding three parts of brown material to one part of green. The bottom layer should always be brown; add a few layers of paper and leaves to the bottom. Next, add a layer of soil between each brown-green layer. Continue this process, following the 3:1 brown-to-green ratio, until you have no more scraps left. The layering and ratio are important to provide the exact amounts of carbon and nitrogen to the compost and to nourish and enrich it.

Sprinkle some water over the layers and cover your compost bin. Keep checking on it every week, sprinkling water, and mixing it. If it starts to smell rotten, add more brown material. Compost generally does not go bad; it is a decomposition process, so it can sometimes smell bad or rotten. Smell does not mean it has gone bad; it just means it is too wet. Add in as much brown material as you feel necessary; however, adding too much can just slow down the decomposition process.

Repeat this same process every week, and it should be ready in about a month or two. Depending on the size of material you use, this can sometimes take longer. Citrus peels for example, take longer to decompose, so if you used these in your compost, expect it to take three or more months.

You will know it's ready when it starts to smell fresh, like the earth on a rainy day. You will no longer be able to see a lot of waste material, as they all will have decomposed to provide nourished soil.

Composting is a slow process. The materials take quite a bit of time to decompose, but the result is a soil that has so many benefits! You can prepare as much compost as you need and use it as an addition to any kind of soil in any plant you are growing.

Growing and Planting Herbs

In order to start an herb garden, there are certain steps you will have to follow to ensure your plants grow well. Every single step, from selecting your seed and sowing it up until the harvest, is crucial and needs to be done with lots of care.

Keep in mind some basic pointers before you start your garden. Some varieties of plants, like thyme, do well in the winter if grown indoors, while others might not survive. It's important that you check and maintain the proper conditions for each plant to ensure you have fresh herbs year-round.

The steps below will explain the process of starting an herb garden and how to maintain it.

Step 1: Planting Seeds

When you go to the store and buy a pack of herb seeds, you will see instructions on the back label. These instructions will give you information on when to sow your seeds, the watering instructions, how much sunlight it needs, and how tall the plant will grow. All this information is specific to each type of herb or plant. Following these instructions carefully will ensure they stay healthy.

When you sow a seed in wet or moist soil, it does not need much water in the first few days. Too much water can cause the seed to drown in the soil. Young plants are very delicate and can break easily; watering too much can destroy them. Just sprinkle water lightly every day until you see it start to sprout and grow into a small seedling. This could take a few days or weeks; information about this will be provided on the label.

Germination trays or seed trays are generally small and made up of plastic, paper, or silicone. They have holes at the bottom to allow water drainage and make it easier for you to sow your seeds. Once they are old enough, you can transfer them to a bigger pot.

1. Add soil or cocopeat (a byproduct of processing coconut) to each section of the germination tray.

2. Sprinkle water on each section to make sure the soil is moist.

3. With a pen or a small gardening tool, make a hole about two centimeters deep in each tray.

4. Gently place two or three seeds in the hole in each section and cover it with a little soil.

5. Sprinkle some more water and allow this to sit in a warm place until it starts to sprout.

Herb seeds usually need a warm place to germinate, so if it is not that warm outside, you can put your plant indoors until it starts to sprout. You can alternatively cover it with a plastic bag, leaving some air holes at the top to keep the heat and moisture in.

Once your seeds are sown, do not try to move or mix the soil, as this can cause the seeds to sink. Also, don't overcrowd a plant pot with too many seeds; always sow lightly to avoid plant crowding. Leave some room between each seed so it has enough space to grow.

Alternatively, you can buy fresh seedlings directly from the store and replant them; skip the first two steps and go directly to step three. When you buy seedlings, the store will have already done most of the initial hard work for you, from planting to maintaining the right environment for germination. You just have to bring them home, repot the young plants, and keep on watering.

Step 2: Keep on Watering

It's important to keep checking on your plants and watering them every day, no matter how young or old they are. A few days after sowing, you will see it start to sprout. Once it sprouts, you can start using a watering can to gently water the soil. Slowly, they start to grow into seedlings. Seedlings are still very young plants but are more well established than sprouts are. You will see a delicate green stem with just a few leaves on it. Maintaining temperature and sunlight becomes more important at this stage.

Just like us humans, plants need a certain temperature to be able to survive. While we can wear a jacket when it gets too cold, plants cannot. The root can freeze if it is too cold, and the plant dies. To avoid this, try to store your seedling in a place where it gets enough heat; however, too much heat is a problem again; the plant gets thirsty and will wilt.

If you are worried about your plants outside, indoor gardens make growing herbs much easier since the temperature can be manually controlled. Move your germination tray indoors, being careful not to disturb the plant, and put it in a warm corner.

Continue to water it every day, and soon you will see your seedling grow into a young plant that is a few inches high.

Step 3: Transferring Young Plants

Now that your plants are a few inches high, their roots need to go deeper into the soil, and the plant needs more space to grow. You now need to transfer your young plant into a bigger pot.

First, get your big pot ready. Make sure there are holes underneath the pot to allow proper drainage. Add the garden soil up to about three-fourths full. With your hands or any other digging tools, make a hole about 6 inches deep in the soil that is in this pot.

Gently remove the plant from the germination tray. You need to be extremely cautious here. The plant is delicate, and some types of movements can damage it. Do not try to pull the plant by its stem or root. Instead, hold it by the complete block of soil and remove the entire contents of each section of the germination tray.

Put this into the hole in the bigger pot, and pack it tightly with some more soil. Alternatively, you can use compost to add more nutrients to your soil. For three cups of garden soil, add one cup of compost—just take an estimate of the quantity; there is no need to be accurate with the ratio here—and mix well.

Water your plant immediately after repotting. This allows it to adjust and feel safe in its new home. Keep a close eye on your plants for a few days after transferring. Sometimes plants stop growing after they are transferred to bigger pots; they need some extra care.

Step 4: Hardening Off Plants for Outdoors

This means to "toughen up" your plants. Your plants were adapted to indoor environments, where they were planted under controlled air, heat, and other factors. Suddenly taking it outside and leaving it there can shock the plant. This concept is like your toddler's first day of daycare; the caretakers would ask you to go along with the kid for a few days until they adjust to the unique environment.

The best time to begin the process of hardening plants is about a week or two before you completely shift them outdoors. Each day, when it is warm, place your plant in a shady spot, like under a tree, where it would still get some sun, but not too much. After sunset, or before it gets dark, bring your plants outside. The idea here is to make your plant adjust to the temperatures outside but bring them back inside at night when it gets too cold.

Leave the plant outside for an increased number of hours each day. If you leave it outside for four hours on the first day, go for five hours on the next. If it's too windy or cold outside, skip putting your plants out on that day.

After a week or two of doing this, your plant is ready for life outside!

Watering Tips!

When it comes to watering plants, there are a few tips that keep your soil healthy and your plants well fed. Plants heavily depend on moisture for their survival, so keeping the soil evenly moist can help promote plant growth.

All plants love water, and herb plants are no exception! Place your herb plant along with its pot in a bowl of water; this creates a water reservoir and allows it to absorb as much water as it needs. The holes at the bottom of the pot will allow the water to flow in or out depending on when it needs it, so this technique even minimizes effort. Self-watering pots work on this same concept—most plants do well in them—so you can consider investing in one to take care of your plants for you.

If you want to manually water your plants, though, do a few quick checks before watering each day:

- Is the top layer of soil moist? If yes, dig a little deeper to make sure the layers inside are not too wet.

- Is there water on the plate underneath? If there is, check the soil again to make sure you are not overwatering your plant.

- Are there yellow or brown leaves? If yes, be sure to cut the leaf off with gardening scissors to ensure the rest of your plant gets a proper supply of water.

Always focus on the root of the plant while watering. The leaves and stem need little to no water. The root absorbs water and keeps your plant healthy, so be sure to maintain proper levels of water in the soil. How often and how much water each plant needs will be discussed in the next session.

Water in the Morning

The time you water your plants, whether morning or evening, actually plays an important role in how well your plant grows. When you water your plants early in the morning, it takes quite a few hours of sunlight for the water to actually get absorbed into their roots.

When you water in the evening, the water tends to rest inside the soil and stay there, causing the root to drown or rot.

Afternoon watering, on the other hand, might not be as effective either. When the sun is too hot, water tends to evaporate before it reaches the root. When it looks like the water is evaporating, you naturally tend to water it more. This results in the plant taking in more water than it actually needs.

Water When You See Dry Soil

When it's too hot outside, your plants feel the same way you do. The top layer of the soil starts to dry and starts to crack. This is a sign that your plants are thirsty and that they need more water. If the top layer is dry and when you mix the soil, it is still dry inside, it is a sign of "plant dehydration." This means that you will need to water your plants more often until the soil starts to show signs of moisture again.

Mix the soil gently without disturbing the roots before you water plants that have dried out. This ensures that the soil absorbs the water and does not just run out.

If possible, try tying your plants to a less sunny spot on days with extreme temperatures; of course, this does affect the aesthetics of your garden, but plant health always comes first.

Fertilizer Water

This might sound a little silly because fertilizer is one thing and water is something else. Did you know that you can create your own non-chemical fertilizer and water your plant while also providing the plant with essential nutrients? Below is a list of a few household food items and scraps that can make great natural fertilizers for all your indoor and outdoor garden plants.

Coffee Fertilizer

Once you drink your coffee, instead of throwing the used coffee grounds away, try putting them to good use. Place them in water overnight, and the next morning, use this to water the leaves of plants in your herb garden. This is a great method of "foliar fertilizing." Foliar fertilizing means directly applying or spraying the fertilizer on the plants' leaves, and not to the root.

Banana Peels

After you finish your banana, take the peel, and put it in a large mason jar. If you don't have one, any dish with a lid is okay. Fill the jar up with water and leave it there for about 48 hours, and then water your plants with peel water. Banana peels contain high amounts of potassium, which is a mineral widely required by plants.

These fertilization methods can also revive a dull-looking plant and make it vibrant, happy, and healthy!

Rice Water

If you are someone who cooks and eats a lot of rice, you know that you need to wash your rice before cooking it. The next time you wash your rice, though, don't let all that nutrient-rich water go into the drain. Instead, collect the water and store it in a separate dish. Use this water to water your plants.

How Often to Water?

Here are a few key points that will help you determine the water needs of your plant.

Plant	Watering Schedule
Basil	Once a week
Chives	Once or twice a week
Cilantro	Every two days, light watering
Dill	Soil always needs to be damp.
Fennel	Everyday
Oregano	Once every two days, allow the soil to dry completely before watering.

Parsley	Once or twice a week
Rosemary	Once a week, provide more sunlight than water.
Thyme	Once every eight or ten days

Keep in mind that if your plants are outdoors, skip watering on rainy days and count this as a watering day. Most herbs, except thyme, require the soil to be damp but not too wet.

Each plant is different; there is no "one size fits all" technique. They need special care, and while it may seem like a bit of work, gardens are worth the time you spend.

Signs of Over and Under Watering

If you start to notice some yellow leaves or wilting leaves, chances are that you are overwatering your plants. This, however, is also a sign of underwatering. So, how do you know the difference?

Check the soil. If it looks too soggy, stop watering your plants and allow them to get some more sun to absorb all that excess water. You might also start to notice a rotten or foul smell coming from the soil. This is an indicator of rotting roots.

Also check the base of the root stem. This should not feel soggy or tough. If it is, you might have overwatered it. Another obvious sign is bacteria or fungus growth on the soil inside your pot.

These signs do not show up overnight—unless it's wet soil—but sometimes take a few days of constant overwatering.

Sunlight Needs

Just like a plant needs water, it also needs sunlight. Even if your herb garden is indoors, it does need to be in an area that gets a few hours of sun each day to stay healthy.

Different Plants and Their Sunlight Requirements

Herbs can be classified into the following types based on their sunlight needs:

- semi-shade herbs

- full-sun herbs

More information on each type is given below.

Semi-Shade Plants

Some herbs will accept semi-shade, which means about three to six hours of sunlight a day. Here is a list of some of these herbs:

- bay leaves

- tarragon

- chervil

- angelica

- parsley

- mint

- coriander

These plants are relatively easy to maintain in urban areas or home gardens since there is a lot of light obstruction due to buildings.

Full-Sun Herbs

The most popular herbs fall into this category. Full sun does not mean that it needs 24 hours of sunlight to grow well—that would make growing it impossible! These herbs need over 6 hours of sunlight a day, so placing them facing east will ensure they get a few hours of that morning sun before the sun is high and houses, trees, and other buildings bring shade.

- basil

- rosemary

- sage

- thyme

- oregano

- mint

- chamomile

- lavender

- parsley

- bay

- coriander

- tarragon

You may notice from the two lists above that there are some herbs listed under both partial and semi-shade. These herbs are exceptionally low maintenance. They can survive well in any condition, low sunlight or full, making them easier to grow than other herbs.

Types of Sun

Yes, the "type" of sun does have a direct effect on plant growth. The morning sun is much cooler and less intense when compared to the afternoon or evening sun. Placing your plants facing a direction where it gets too many hours of afternoon sun and little or no morning sun can exhaust them and cause them to wilt.

To understand the type of sun your herb needs, check the label of the packaging that your seeds came in. This will have detailed instructions on how much sun it needs, classifying it into various types. You may see one of the following:

- full sun—six or more hours a day

- light shade—three to five hours a day

- partial shade—two to three hours a day

- full shade—one hour a day

- dense shade—no direct sunlight

While there is a category for dense shade, almost none of the regular herbs can survive with no direct sunlight.

Too Much or Too Little Sun: What Happens?

Too much or too little of anything never did anyone any good. It works the same way with plants. Too much sun can cause the leaves of the plant to turn yellow. Plants can get sunburned too, and turning yellow is their way of showing you that their placement is not right.

When a plant gets too little sun, that is a bigger problem. There is a risk of your herbs underperforming and eventually dying. Chlorophyll is a pigment that gives the plant its green color, and when your plant does not get the sun it needs, it does not produce chlorophyll, causing it to turn yellow. When you see a leaf turn yellow, don't worry. It doesn't have to be the end of your plant's life. You can still save it! Move it to a place that gets a little less sun and cut off the yellow leaves. Continue to water it well, and it should be back in a few weeks!

Artificial Lights

There are quite a few reasons why home gardens, especially in urban areas, might not get enough sunlight. Maybe your house is facing south, or there are other buildings blocking the sunlight, or the area where you want your garden to be is not at an angle that gets even a little sun.

Don't let this be the reason you can't grow your own herbs. Artificial lights or grow lights are always an option. Artificial lighting replicates the natural sun and provides the heat and light a plant would need. These are designed for indoor gardens and can fit quite well in small spaces.

There is one special type of basil called *holy basil*, which is native to India. It is known for its high medicinal value. A holy basil tea can cure colds and improve breathing. It can also be used in soups for the same reason. You can find this herb around the world, although it isn't as readily available. If you do manage to find some, though, place it in an area that gets full sunlight. Since India is a tropical country, herbs native to that region will need to have artificial or natural conditions mimicking their home. In the winter, bring the plant indoors to make sure it survives. For this kind of plant, artificial lights work wonders at keeping it alive for the next seasons.

What's so impressive about these grow lights is that they allow you to grow any herbs—not just holy basil—all year round! That includes even the darkest winter days when the temperature is less than -5° F outside! Imagine a nice, hot bowl of tomato soup with some home-grown thyme on top after a long day at work in that kind of weather! That right there is motivation for you to grow your own herbs and get that artificial lighting!

Small grow lights can be placed almost everywhere, even in small places. Some tests (The 12 Best Grow Lights of 2024, Tested and Reviewed, 2024) show that these lights even help plants grow better than natural sunlight! The best part is that basic lights are not even as expensive as you would think! Some are priced as low as $30 US, making them a perfect and affordable investment!

Chapter 3:

Gathering Your Bounty—How to

Harvest and Store Herbs

In just a few months of providing it with love and care, you will have a beautiful-looking garden that is full of healthy herbs! Give yourself a pat on the back. You did an amazing job planting and maintaining your garden! The next step is harvesting your herbs. There are some specific rules and guidelines related to when, where, and how to trim your plants to ensure they keep growing for the next season.

Harvesting Herbs

When to Trim and Where to Trim?

I know it might seem like a difficult task to do. You have a beautiful-looking plant that you took care of, and now you just must cut it up. But the whole reason you have an herb garden is to be able to use the herbs for the benefit of your health and to add flavor to your food. Also, by trimming the grown stems, you are helping the plant grow happier and healthier too! Here are a few trimming tips below:

1. Always cut or trim your herbs with clean and sharp gardening scissors.

2. Don't cut stems when they are too old.

3. Each herb needs to be cut in a specific way to ensure it grows more leaves.

Oregano and thyme, however, are much simpler for a beginner to trim. You don't need to worry at all about them, and you can pretty much cut them on any stem or in any direction. Both of these herbs will still continue to grow leaves in the trimmed area. They also tend to spread across wide areas, so try to trim the edges to ensure they stay confined to their spots.

Here are some simple instructions on trimming different types of herbs, including chives, sage, parsley, cilantro, rosemary, dill, mint, lavender, and bay leaves.

To trim chives, cut half an inch above the soil for each stem. For sage, leave a few leaves at the base and cut the stem above.

Parsley grows back well when trimmed close to the base, about an inch or two from the soil.

When cutting or pruning cilantro, start cutting the leaves when the plant is about six inches tall in sunny areas to prevent flowering and encourage strong regrowth.

Dill is a relatively short-lived plant. Cut the stem close to the soil, leaving an inch from the base to prevent flowering.

Mint can be harvested from any point. It keeps growing, growing, and growing more, so be sure you give it its own container to be sure it does not grow over other plants.

For lavender, cut the stem above the leaves. Lavender also goes through a growth spurt, where it can overgrow, especially during the summer.

For bay leaves, you can handpick or trim the leaves. It's best to remove the larger leaves first.

For rosemary, some types grow long, woody stems that can be used in grilling to add flavor. Cut off the stem and just pop it into the grill along with your meat to give it an enhanced flavor. If your plant has stems like this, cut them about an inch above the soil to be able to use them and get extra flavor from the complete stem. Rosemary can be pruned at any height or from any part of the plant and will regrow well; just be sure not to damage the root. The plant tends to overgrow in some seasons, so heavy trimming might be necessary during harvest season or in the fall.

The bottom line for trimming is to cut off as much as you can once it's ready and before it starts to flower. Herbs don't last long after they flower, so cut them early since the aim is to give plants a long life.

How to Trim?

Now that you know the exact spot you need to trim each of your herbs, there is one last step before you can actually go and start the process. How do you trim your herbs? Just like humans, plants take some time for their cuts to heal. Messy cuts can take much longer to heal than precise ones, allowing the possibility of disease.

Always make cuts at an angle to prevent the water from sitting on the plant's open wound. This minimizes the risk of water droplets being able to settle on it. Also, as another crucial step, wash or disinfect your gardening scissors prior to trimming so that no bacteria enter the plant when you prune.

If it's important to you to make sure the plant still looks aesthetically pleasing even after trimming, be sure to maintain a balance of cut stems on all sides. Take a step back from your plant and make sure everything looks even.

Always remember that with herbs, the more you trim, the more they will grow. Keep on trimming to make sure your plant grows bigger and better!

Drying and Storing Herbs

Sometimes, your herb plant grows so much before you even realize it that it needs to be trimmed. That leaves you with too many herbs ready to harvest and not enough food to cook before they spoil. Now you could cut up some stems and give them to your neighbors or friends, but if you choose to keep them for yourself, drying is a great way to make herbs last longer.

There are so many ways to dry your herbs. Some people like to tie them up and leave them in the oven for a while until they're dry and crisp. This is one way of doing it, but there are a few other ways you can try as well. You can use whichever method is easier for you.

I know it might seem like if you are drying them anyway, you can just get them from the store. But the main advantage here is that you know they are fresh. The ones in supermarkets might be a little older and not freshly dried. This reduces their shelf life to much less than that of homemade dried herbs.

You saw in the previous section how to dry herbs to make tea. There are, however, a few more guidelines you need to follow to ensure that your dried herbs last longer and stay fresh. If properly dried and stored, herbs can stay fresh for about one or two years!

Trimming

The first step to drying herbs is trimming them. For each herb, there is a specific way to trim it, all of which you have seen in the earlier section.

If you plan to dry herbs tomorrow, make sure you freshly pick them on the morning of the same day to make sure they are fresh. If they are a few days old and stored in the refrigerator, some leaves might have already turned brown or black, reducing their shelf life after drying. That completes step one of the drying processes.

For herbs like rosemary, sage, thyme, and parsley, you would have them close to the stem, as seen in the table above. This makes it easier to air-dry them in small bunches.

Cleaning

Once you trim your bunch of herbs, set them on your kitchen counter or someplace else. Take a good look at the leaves, and make sure they do not contain any spoilt areas, dark colored areas, and so on.

Also, remove any dirt or soil residue from the trimmings. Most importantly, make sure there are no insects residing in the plant. This step is important to make sure your herb doesn't spoil or go bad once it is dried.

Once they are cleaned and prepared, you can now go on to select a method of drying.

Methods of Drying Herbs

Air Drying

Less tender herbs, like rosemary, sage, thyme, and parsley, are best when they are airdried. Start by creating a small bunch of each individual herb. Now, wrap the ends of each bunch with a piece of yarn or thread, making sure you secure the bunch well. Make sure there is no moisture in your bunch of herbs, since it can cause them to rot. This is also a reason the bunch needs to be kept small to allow air circulation.

Using the other end of the thread, suspend the herbs from a clothesline using a clip. This is best done indoors, in a well-ventilated but not too sunny area.

Other herbs, like basil, oregano, and mint, tend to retain a lot of moisture. For that reason, we need to add an additional step before we hang them to dry. Pat the herbs with a dry kitchen towel. Now, punch some holes in a paper bag and form a bouquet. Now, put smaller bunches in each paper bag and secure the whole thing well. You can hang it to dry like you did for the other herbs.

This method takes a bit of time, and you will know they are ready when they start to crumble as soon as you touch them.

Dehydrator Drying

If you have a food dehydrator, it makes things much easier. You can dry herbs in bulk, and you can do it quickly! Set them in a single layer on each tray of your dehydrator. Set it to the lowest setting and leave your herbs there for about two or three hours.

Once done, you can remove them and prepare them for storage. Sometimes, though, with a dehydrator, you see that some bits are stuck to the tray and are hard to remove. Gently tap to pull these off carefully so that there is no waste.

Microwave Drying

Drying your herbs in the microwave generally does work but is not recommended as much as the other methods. Some microwaves heat up too fast and can destroy your herb instead of drying it.

If you can, though, set a small amount of your herbs in a single layer on a clean piece of paper. Put this in the microwave, and microwave for 30 seconds. Check your herbs, mix them, and put them in for another 30 seconds. Repeat this process for about two or three minutes, depending on your microwave. Always keep an eye on them, and if you notice any smells, stop the process immediately, and turn off your microwave.

Sun Drying

Sun drying is an easy and natural way to preserve herbs. You can do this on your own patio or balcony. Choose a warm, sunny day to dry your herbs. It takes a day or two for them to completely dry, and you need to plan this in advance, so a weather or forecast app can help you with this.

To dry them, spread out the herbs in an even layer on a clean plate, cloth, or anything else that is convenient for you, and just leave them in a nice, sunny spot.

Sun-dried herbs help retain their natural flavor and aroma. It is a cost-effective method—it literally costs you nothing! Also, if you are someone who is concerned about energy usage, sun drying is perfect for you! Just as a small tip, avoid drying herbs in direct sunlight for prolonged periods, as it may cause them to lose their color and flavor.

Oven Drying

Arrange your leaves in a single layer on a silicone baking sheet or muslin cloth. These work better than a baking tray and prevent herbs from sticking to them. When that is done, preheat your oven to about 80°F and put the herbs in for about 10 minutes.

Take them out to check on them; give them a little mix. This ensures they get enough air and don't stick to the tray. Then, put them back in the oven again. Depending on the thickness of the leaves and how big they are, they should be completely dry in about 25 to 30 minutes.

Remember to keep checking on them and turn the oven off as soon as they are crispy and crumbly. Over-drying the herbs can cause them to lose their flavor and they won't be as fun to use in dishes. Sometimes, it can also result in a burnt flavor, which overpowers the food's taste.

Storing the Dried Herbs

In any method you choose to follow, you will know your herbs are dried when they crumble to the touch and look crisp. There are multiple ways to keep your herbs fresh:

- Avoid exposure to air, light, and heat.

- store in a refrigerator or freezer.

- store in a dark, dry place.

If you store your herbs in a refrigerator, make sure they are stored in an airtight container and that you take only as much as you need to use out of the container and immediately put the box back inside. When it thaws, it might start to form excess moisture, causing it to rot.

Glass jars or mason jars are other options that work well to store your dried herbs.

You can also put the dried herb in a blender and make a powder out of it. Check that the blender is clean and dry before putting your herb in it. You can store it in the same way and use half a teaspoon—or more or less—in any recipe you want to. Powder is also much easier to incorporate into soups and stews.

You can also create your own herb rub for seasoning pork chops, lamb or steak. Combine a few powdered herbs and add some dried spices to rub onto your meat. You have access to a variety of different herbs right in your garden, so feel free to explore new flavor combinations. Most herbs work well together and complement each flavor.

Labelling Containers

Labeling is an important part of storage. Make sure you label correctly to avoid surprises when you cook your food! You don't want your soup to taste like cilantro when you were expecting to flavor it with thyme! Labeling also makes it easier for anyone who is cooking to find what they need.

On the label, add the date you dried and stored them so you can determine how fresh they are. Your fridge will look more organized as well, and you'll know when an herb needs to be restocked.

Storing Fresh Herbs

Most fresh herbs need to be stored in the refrigerator; when stored properly, they last for a few weeks. Here are a few tips on how you can keep each herb fresh and ready for use when you need it.

Firstly, washing and cleaning your herbs before you store them is important, as it can help prevent pests and other insects from internally spoiling your herbs. No matter what herb you choose to store, make sure you clean it thoroughly before starting the storage process.

For herbs like basil, wash them thoroughly and pat them dry with a clean kitchen towel. Place them on the countertop in a cool place away from direct sunlight.

For the others, like oregano, cilantro, and parsley, store them in the refrigerator. Fill a jar or glass of water about two or three inches high. Place a small bunch of your herbs, stem first, into the water. Make sure none of the stems touch the water. Place a plastic bag above the bunch to keep it fresh.

Alternatively, you can wrap your herb bundle in a paper towel and set it on a refrigerator rack. This way, they last fresh for quite a few days.

Storing Plants for Longevity

We know that we can dry the herbs after cutting or trimming to ensure they stay for a longer time. But, for some herbs, known as perennial plants, you can save the entire plant through the seasons to ensure that it grows back again after the last frost date in the spring. These will be discussed in further detail in the next chapter, but now let's take a look at a few techniques that will come in handy to store plants for longevity.

If you are growing plants outside in pots or growing them directly into garden beds, bringing them indoors is a good option to help them withstand different seasons and extreme weather.

To do this, gently transfer your plants from the garden beds into a container or pot with soil. Slowly start to bring them into places that get some shade during the day. This means you would start by putting it in a sunny spot for a few hours each day and then bringing it onto the porch or another shady spot for the rest of the day. Gradually reduce the amount of time it spends outside before completely bringing it indoors.

Once it is ready to be completely switched indoors, clean the plant and it's leaves thoroughly with water to ensure there are no bugs, dust, or other pests in the soil that might enter your home.

Place the plant close to your window or under an artificial light to ensure its longevity. Remember, your herb plant needs some sun, so use these grow lights if you can't find a place that can get at least a few hours of sunlight each day.

Once indoors, the plants will need less water, so water them less often than you did while they were outside.

Mulching

If you want to leave your plants outside during the winter, you may be able to do so, but you will need to take some extra precautions to ensure your plant doesn't die in the dark and cold days. One way to protect them is called mulching.

Step one is choosing the right mulch for the winter. What is mulch? Mulch is a material that is laid over soil to cover it and help preserve the moisture in the soil to make it fit for different climate conditions. It works as an insulation layer and protects the plant's roots from both extreme high and low temperatures.

There are a lot of different types of mulch, so be sure to consider your individual needs before buying one. During winter, for example, hay or straw mulch is used to protect the roots and soil from frost. For the summer, on the other hand, gravel or grass clippings are more preferred since they can keep the soil cool and the moisture in.

If you have a large garden, consider getting a contract from companies that offer professional mulching services, to avoid potential problems or damage to your soil.

For winters, always mulch after your area's first frost date and before the earth starts to freeze. It's important not to over mulch since this can create a home for unwanted pests and rodents. A three-to four-inch layer should be enough to keep your plants protected.

For summer, apply your mulch layer after the season's last frost date, or when the ground starts to get too hot.

How do you identify the first and last frost date? Just like the names sound, the first frost date is the date in winter when the risk of your plants freezing starts to go high. The temperatures in the winter make life for most plants difficult, and they need a lot of care during this time to help them last until the next season.

The last frost date, on the other hand, is the exact opposite. The risk of plants dying during frost is reduced and continues to decrease as spring progresses. These dates are specific to each region and country, and outdoor plants are generally planted after the season's last frost date. Even within the US, for example, the frost dates in Denver are different from those in Austin, Los Angeles, or New York. You can find a lot of information on the internet about your specific region and its average frost dates.

Predictions for frost dates are not one hundred percent accurate, and they might come a week before or after; there are no specific signs to indicate this exactly. Most importantly, there is no rule that you need to start planting exactly on that particular day.

Tarp Cover

Tarp covers are another effective method to keep your plant's roots warm and protected through extreme weather conditions. Plastic covers are one way to cover your plants, but they usually aren't recommended as they do not allow room for your plant to breathe. If you do choose to use them, allow enough space between the stems and the cover to make sure the plant does not suffocate and rot. Tarp covers made of natural materials, like cotton and linen, are best for your plants.

Waterproof poly tarps are another good option for your plants and are easily available in stores online or at other hardware stores.

Avoid Pruning or Fertilizing in Winter

Plants need to be well maintained throughout all other seasons of the year to ensure they stay strong and healthy in the winter. Any activity related to plants, like pruning or fertilizing, needs to be done during these other seasons; doing this in the winter can actually be harmful to them.

When you prune plants, especially herbs, in the winter, they might not grow back. The internal part of the plant is exposed and cannot heal. This attracts insects and diseases in the later months.

Chapter 4:

Using Your Harvest—Cooking and

Experimenting with Herbs

Gardening is a long process, but it never gets boring! And when your herbs are ready for harvest, the flavor that they add to your dishes makes it worth all that effort!

In this chapter, you will learn all about what your herbs can do and where and when to use them, not just in the kitchen but also as medicine. Additionally, you can make a natural fertilizer out of herbs that not only smells good but is healthy for you and your plants too! Inhaling chemicals and sending them out into the environment causes a lot of pollution, so natural fertilizers can reverse the effect while still providing room for a healthy environment.

From homemade herbal remedies and natural oils for hair growth to lotions and skin care routines, the possibilities for using herbs are endless. Throughout this chapter, you'll find information on how to use herbs for things you might not have even thought about!

Cooking With Herbs

When you first think of herbs, you think of salads or soups. While both of these are good ways to make use of your herbs, there are quite a few other beginner-friendly ways for you to put your herbs to good use.

Cooking with herbs isn't a skill that you master; it's an art that you understand and interpret. Adding too much of some types of herbs can overpower the dish, but again, this totally depends on the perception of the people eating it. Some find strong tastes unsettling, while others might actually enjoy the same dish. Cooking with herbs is all about finding balance.

Cutting them into really thin pieces can help release the oils and bring out the flavor of the herbs. Always bundle up two or three herb leaves, fold them, and make a few cuts down the center. This makes it easier to cut leaves into smaller pieces.

One key point to remember is that dried herbs can be stronger than fresh herbs. They have a deeper taste, so using a smaller amount of dried herbs than fresh brings about a stronger flavor to the dish.

Herb Salsa

A fresh herb salsa pairs well with any dish! You can add a spoonful—or more—of salsa onto a cup of steamed vegetables, if you are on a diet, or eat them with your seafood, pork, or beef if you're not! It's an amazing way to make even the simplest of dishes taste so fresh, light, and delicious!

Herb salsa Verde is also so simple to make and includes just a few simple ingredients: herbs of your choice, olive oil, lemon, salt, pepper, and some garlic! All you need to do is blend everything together in a food processor and use it as dressing!

Salsa fresca, or *Pico de Gallo,* is another simple Mexican salsa that you can make using cilantro, tomato, white onion, and jalapeño.

Gravy With Herbs

Serving a rich gravy alongside any roast—duck, turkey, chicken, and more—can make it extra special, especially when it is served hot.

Once you are done cooking and roasting your bird, you can use the juices from the roasting tray to make a gravy just by adding herbs, and a few simple ingredients. Add the roasting juices to a tray with onion, tomato, parsley, rosemary, and thyme. Pour in chicken stock and cook for a while. Sieve and serve with your roast! Make this gravy to pair with any holiday roast, and it will be a highlight dish for all your guests!

Salad Dressing

An olive oil and vinegar-based vinaigrette is so easy to make and can elevate all kinds of salads to make them more enjoyable. Even if you aren't a "salad person," the flavor and aroma of this dressing will make you want to try it.

It is so simple to make and allows room for as much customization as you like! Feel free to experiment with different flavors and herbs by adding more of this and less of that and soon, you'll have created your own perfect recipe for a flavorful vinaigrette! Share it with others, and when they ask where you got the idea from, you can proudly say that it's your own!

There is no strict ratio or recipe for this type of salad dressing, so if you don't like oil, add less of it; if you love it, add more. It will not negatively affect the taste.

Once made, you can also store it in the fridge for a few days. It works well with all kinds of salads; just be sure to toss your salad after adding in the dressing to ensure every bit is covered with flavor from that vinaigrette.

Pasta Sauce

Everyone loves good pasta, right? Did you know that you can incorporate different herbs into your pasta sauce, not just oregano? Parsley, basil, thyme, cilantro, and chives are all excellent flavorful herbs that can elevate any kind of sauce. Add in minced garlic too, fry everything up a little, and in no time, you'll have the perfect pasta that is the star of any dinner party! You can even use a jar of canned sauce as the base for your pasta sauce, add in a few herbs, and no one will ever know it's premade!

If you want to stay simple and take the original route, though, you have some oregano growing in your garden too!

Meat Marinade

Marinating is one of the most important steps to cooking your meat, or tofu, if you are vegan. Prepare your marinade in a large bowl with olive oil, basil, thyme, rosemary, tarragon, chive, and any other herb you want to use.

For more flavor and seasoning, add in some garlic, salt, and pepper, and allow your meat to soak in this marinade for a few hours before you begin to cook it. This will definitely make a difference to the overall flavor, making it taste "five-star" style.

One of the best parts about using an herb marinade is that you can use as many or as few herbs as you like! Allow yourself to get creative with different flavors and bring something new to the table each day. That way, dinner never gets boring!

Side Dishes

Along with your protein, you might want to serve up some sides, like roasted potatoes or tomatoes. They make a great addition to any main course, especially when made with flavorful herbs. You can use herbs to flavor your side dishes to make them taste just as great as your protein does! You will *want* to eat and finish your portion of vegetables for the day. This is a clever idea to get kids to eat their greens! Broccoli tots flavored with some herbs make a great lunch box side dish or snack that they will enjoy! Simply steam some broccoli along with some potatoes, mash well with a fork, and add in some salt and pepper. Add a small amount of fresh herbs, mix, roll, and shape with a cookie cutter, and serve!

If you are looking for other ideas for side dishes, cherry tomatoes, basil, and mozzarella cheese make a great skewer that goes perfectly with any meat or as an appetizer. Herbs don't just need to be used in combination with meat; here are a few vegan dishes that you can make with herbs.

- herb quinoa with lemon

- grilled eggplant with an herb vinaigrette

- sweet potato fries with herb dip

- cauliflower steak with herbal balsamic dressing

- zucchini fries with herb batter.

To make an herb batter for your zucchini fries, add in a cup of flour and make a regular batter. Now add in some fresh and dried herbs of your choice and give it another mix. Dip your zucchini into the batter and deep-fry it until golden! You can do the same with potatoes, sweet potatoes, or even carrots!

Dessert

This might sound like an odd or weird combination at first. Who eats ice cream with basil, right? It is actually the perfect summer sweet treat! Try it by taking a scoop of vanilla ice cream and topping it up with some strawberry or raspberry jam. Then add some finely chopped basil on top! You can also create layers of jam, ice cream, and basil to create a family-sized tub that you can enjoy over a movie!

This hits you with a burst of flavor, and the versatility of this dessert concept allows room for as much customization as you want. Drizzle some chocolate syrup over your berry and basil-infused ice cream. This adds another spin on the already unique taste. You can also dip your ice cream cone in some crushed or powdered nuts on top for that added texture and crunch.

An herb and feta cheese pie might sound like it won't taste good, but it actually does! Most people, when they think of a dessert, think of sweets, chocolate, and fruit. At any regular bakery or store, you might not see a lot of herbal pies. But once you try it, you just keep craving more. Pies are simple to make, unlike cake, and taste really good! The next time you invite friends or family over for dinner, use a cup of herbs from your garden—fresh herbs work best for pies—and incorporate them into your pie crust or filling.

Cocktail

You might have seen mint being used in a lot of cocktails. It adds a really nice flavor and aroma to the drink. Other herbs can be used to complement cocktails as well, like basil, rosemary, elderflower, and others. During Christmas, try a winter rosemary sangria!

When it comes to making herb-infused cocktails, the varieties and options are endless, so get your creative juices flowing! With freshly picked herbs from your garden, you can create endless types of cocktails—lavender lemonade, mint vodka, cranberry and thyme gin, and so many more. When you host a party or get-together, you will even have your own special bar at home that has the most unique drinks! Pair this with some herb-infused meat, and people will be talking about that party for ages!

You'll have unique drinks for each season: spicy drinks for the fall, bright drinks for the summer, and flavorful drinks for the winter.

Fresh Herbal Tea

Herbal teas—we have seen a lot about them in an earlier chapter. Just take a spoonful of your dry herbs and allow them to infuse in a cup of hot water for about five minutes. They taste great, and they also give you a sense of relaxation.

Some teas are even proven (Mechanisms Underlying the Anti-Depressive Effects of Regular Tea Consumption, 2019) to be able to reduce the risk of depression. Herbal tea culture is especially popular in Germany, and they believe teas can have a soothing effect when incorporated into daily routines. Here are a few ideas:

- fresh chamomile tea

- lavender tea

- mint tea

- basil and mint tea

- rosemary tea

- lemon balm

Herb Butter

Herb butter is one of the simplest things you can make, and it goes well with toast, garlic bread, pasta, Indian food, and lots of other foods as well!

It also stays fresh for about a week in the refrigerator and about a month in the fridge, so it's okay to pre-make your herb butter to make cooking dinner simpler and much more flavorful!

All you have to do is take some butter and allow it to warm up to room temperature. Then, add in your favorite herbs such as cilantro, thyme, rosemary, and some salt. Give it a good whisk! It will smell so light and fragrant and can take any dish to a higher level.

Cooking doesn't need to be complex. You don't need to be a chef to cook a delicious meal. Herbs make it easy for anyone to be able to cook a meal and excel!

Beyond the Kitchen

It's not just in cooking; herbs have plenty of uses in self-care as oils, creams, and more. Herbal aromatherapy is a very common method used to promote relaxation, and even help with symptoms of anxiety and depression. Some other areas where herbs come in handy are explained below.

Promoting Hair Growth

Oiling your hair helps it grow really well and gives it a glossy look. It can even help cut down on the frizz! Rosemary has been the trend for quite a while now; rosemary water or oil for hair growth have been all over social media for their numerous benefits. This isn't actually a trend or one of those life hacks that never actually work. It's a proven-to-work natural remedy (Uronnacchi et. al., 2022) that has been around for a few hundred years.

Rosemary-infused argan oil is like "liquid gold" for your hair and can help promote hair growth by strengthening your roots.

You need a lot of rosemary to make this oil, so it's a perfect way to make use of all the excess rosemary that you have during harvest season right before the winter. However, be sure that you dry your herb using one of the methods mentioned earlier to avoid mold forming in your oil.

Homemade Herbal Lipbalm

Those lip balms you get in stores that are "all natural" are way too expensive, right? Think about how much money you could save by making your own chapped lip remedy at home with fresh herbs from your garden! You'll know exactly what's going into it and can be sure it's cruelty-free (if that is something you care about)!

These lip balms take some time to make since we need to make a herbal oil first, but you can customize the color using a little bit—or a lot—of beet powder to go perfectly with your skin tone!

You can use peppermint and lemon balm as herbs to make your lip balm, since they both give that menthol-like cool feeling that most store-bought lip balms have.

Since these are generally made from only natural ingredients like beeswax and oil, Store them in a cool place, like the refrigerator, to make sure they don't melt. You can carry a little box with you in your purse for when you do a light make-up touch-up. Just don't forget the box in your car!

Aromatherapy

Aromatherapy is a very popular technique used to provide a calming effect on a person. To do this at home, you can leave a diffuser on in any room of your house, and it will spread its aroma, causing a calming feeling. Alternatively, you can sit and meditate in a closed room for about fifteen minutes with a light diffuser on. Both meditation and the aroma work together to brighten up your mood and bring a sense of relaxation to your mind.

You can also schedule an appointment with a licensed therapist, who can guide you through the process for a set period of time. They might even give you a massage with a mixture of essential oil and carrier oil. After a session, you will leave feeling calm and relaxed.

If you want to make better use of the herbs you have at home, which is a great practice, you can make your own infusion by simply boiling orange peels with some rosemary. This gives off an earthy smell and fills your home with a fresh scent.

Boiling other herbs, like peppermint and lavender, gives the same therapeutic effect.

Relaxing Baths

Have you ever heard of an herb bath? Lavender is one of the most commonly used herbs to promote relaxation and is the perfect choice for a bath.

Crush some freshly picked lavender in your palm and add it to warm water when you run a bath. This gives a stress-reducing bath experience. Alternatively, you can add half a spoon of dried lavender powder to your bath, and it will have the same effect.

Relax in the warm water for as long as you like, take gentle breaths in and out, and try to focus on the strong smell of lavender.

Peppermint baths also have many benefits and can serve as a detox. Make and store some peppermint bath salts with Epsom salt, dead sea salt, some dried peppermint powder, and a few freshly cut and chopped peppermint leaves. This also makes a great gift for any occasion!

Bug Spray

As fun as summer and spring are, they come with their own problems. A major one is bugs. Lucky for you, your herb garden is full of fresh herbs that can make perfect insect repellents. Mix some witch hazel with water, mint, and lavender to create your own natural bug spray!

Combining witch hazel and peppermint also makes a natural bug spray that can keep you bug-free if you prefer a minty fragrance over the strong smell of lavender.

Basil and chives also have a strong odor that, when used as a spray, can keep flies away from your garden and home.

Propagating Herbs

If you don't want to use your herbs immediately, you have the option of growing more plants from your trimmings! One of the easiest ways to propagate a plant is to cut off a stem from the plant using the general rules previously discussed. Then, put that trimming in a glass of water until it grows roots. Once it does, put it back in the soil, and it will grow into a healthy plant in no time!

To trim the plant, make sure there are some strong leaves on top and that the stem is long enough to fit in a glass of water. It should float around in the glass, and the bottom of the stem should not touch the floor of the glass. This allows space for the roots to grow; if there isn't enough room, the stem will just dry out.

Now, cut off the leaves from the stem, leaving only a few at the top. The idea is that no leaves should be submerged in the glass of water. In about a week, you will see that roots start to appear inside the water. The water level also decreases as the roots grow, so make sure you keep adding water to the glass every day. When the roots are about three or four inches long, remove the stem from the glass and put it back into a pot of soil.

Be sure to harden off your herbs (using the process discussed in Chapter 2) after planting if you plan to keep them outdoors to avoid shock.

For herbs like rosemary, oregano, thyme, and lavender, you can skip the process of glass and water and simply poke the trimming into the soil. These plants can grow roots on their own and propagate. Take care not to move the trimming until the roots are well established. You will know that they are growing well when you start to see fresh green leaves close to and on the stem. Keep on watering like you regularly would.

Chapter 5:

Selecting and Choosing Plants—A

Comprehensive Herb Guide

Now that you know exactly how to plant, grow, harvest, and what to do with each kind of herb, it's time to take a look at some starter herbs that you, even as a total beginner, can successfully grow. Selecting herbs might seem difficult at first; there are so many to choose from and so many uses for each one that you might not know where to start. This chapter breaks down each type of herb and its most common use to make it easy for you to pick what you need.

Let's take a look at the classification of herbs to make things easier to understand. Herbs are mostly of two types: annual and perennial.

Annual herbs are those that complete their life cycle in one year and will have to be planted by seed again the next year. When you see your cilantro plant, for example, wilt and die, don't feel you made a mistake in planting or watering or be sad for not being able to help revive it. It's not your fault at all. Cilantro is an annual herb, and it's wilting just means it has gone through and completed its life cycle for the season. Some more examples of annual herbs are:

- dill

- German chamomile

- chervil

- parsley

- basil

Parsley does classify as an annual plant, but it's a "biennial," which means it stays for two years before it dies. Most people, though, prefer to plant parsley fresh every year from seed, since it's more fresh that way.

Perennial herbs, on the other hand, are much more resilient and can continue to grow through different seasons when given proper care and kept under protected environments. They might seem dormant through the winter, but they are definitely not dead. These plants have the ability to grow back in full bloom in the spring, as long as you keep the roots safe and warm in a cold climate.

In the next season, they will take in all the nutrients from the soil and grow back just as strong as you remember them. Mulching, as we discussed in the earlier chapters, can help protect the plant from harsh weather. A few examples of perennial herbs are

- chives

- mint

- oregano

- rosemary

- tarragon

- thyme

- fennel

- holy basil

- lemongrass

Let's now discuss some of these easy-to-grow herbs in detail, their light and water requirements, and some additional tips to maintain them.

Basil

Basil is one of the easiest herbs to grow and grows rapidly in temperatures ranging from 80° to 90 °F.

Light and Water Requirements

Basil loves the warmth! It can only grow once the weather is hot enough to warm up the soil a little bit. Once the soil is warm and the weather is sunny, basil will grow just about anywhere—in a pot, a windowsill, a garden bed, or in any other sunny spot.

The plant needs about six to eight hours of sunlight each day to be able to grow strong and tall. If that isn't possible, basil can do fine in partial shade too. Keep watching the sun patterns and try to put your basil in a place that gets a lot of sun during the day, especially early in the morning. Once you understand the sun's patterns, you can start growing basil in every sunny corner you have around the house, both indoors and outdoors!

Basil also likes moist soil. Water your plant a few times each week if you are growing indoors. Take care to ensure that the soil does not dry out. The soil always needs to be moist, but not too wet or dry.

Always water your basil plant early in the morning to ensure the roots absorb the moisture well.

The Best Uses of Basil

Did you know that basil can be a great topping for your pizza? Cut a few whole leaves of basil and arrange them on your pizza along with some other toppings for a unique flavor.

Basil also creates a great pasta sauce—no, not just for making pesto! It can be used as a flavoring for your creamy pasta or tomato sauce base.

You can also make a chimichurri and go vegan for your homemade sauce by replacing parmesan with some vegan cheese.

Roasted tomato and basil soup is another idea for dinner that will leave you craving more.

If you are craving Thai food, try some Thai chicken with basil, or basil tofu if you are vegan.

You can also top your salad or sandwich with some finely chopped basil to give it a little bit of freshness.

Additional Tips for Growing and Maintaining Basil

1. Pinch off the topmost leaves once the plant is at least six inches tall to ensure the plant grows taller.

2. Always check the moisture levels in the soil.

3. Trim your plant often to prevent overgrowth.

4. Don't let it flower!

5. Add some compost to your soil to ensure your plant is well fed with all the nutrients it needs.

Chives

Chives are another herb that love the sun. They also prefer about six to eight hours of sun a day, but will do just as well in partial shade. Chives grow beautiful pink flowers, which are also edible!

Light and Water Requirements

Always water your chives deeply so the root gets enough water. Watering once a week should be good enough to ensure chives grow strong and healthy, but always make sure you check their soil; if it seems too dry, water more often.

Whether you are growing chives indoors or outdoors, make sure it gets a few hours of sun each day. In the winter, opt for artificial lighting to ensure the plants survive through the season.

The Best Ways to Use Chives

Chives are the best way to garnish any dish. Make some scrambled eggs and season them with a little salt and pepper. They might taste regular this way, but sprinkling some chives on top gives them an extra special flavor.

They also make a great topping for soups and dips. Another use of this herb is in creating flavorful chive butter, which can then be used to make gravy, toast some bread, or roast your meat and vegetables.

Instead of using regular butter for your garlic bread, use some chive butter for a unique flavor. You can also make a dish as simple as mashed potatoes taste next-level by simply adding a garnish of thinly sliced chives.

Additional Tips for Growing and Maintaining Chives

If you don't want to grow your chives from seeds, you can always regrow them from store-bought chives. Use the propagation techniques from the previous chapters to regrow your store-bought chives.

Make sure you go to the organic produce section of your grocery store and pick up the chives that have bulbs. The bulb is where the root grows when you leave it submerged in water, and without it, the plant will not be able to successfully propagate. Once the roots are well established, put the chives in some soil and ensure the entire bulb is covered and under the soil.

Dill

Outdoor dill is much easier to care for than indoor dill; the reason being its high sunlight requirements. It does do okay with some afternoon shade, but it needs the morning sun in order to thrive.

Light and Water Requirements

Place it in a sunny spot, preferably east-facing spots, where the morning sun is the strongest to ensure proper growth.

Also, make sure there are no tall plants or trees surrounding your dill plant that can block sunlight. As much as dill likes the sun, though, it does not enjoy the heat. Consider applying some mulching techniques to your soil to keep moisture in.

Similar to the other herbs, make sure that you don't water them too much. The soil should be moist but not wet.

If your dill plant is indoors, consider investing in some grow LED lights to mimic the six hours of sun it needs.

The Best Ways to Use Dill

If you like Greek food, you'll know that dill goes well with everything! It has a wide variety of uses in European and Asian dishes, especially in roasted vegetables and meats, soups, and dips like *tzatziki*.

It goes perfectly well with your meat marinade or for pan-seared pork and lamb. If you are vegetarian, toss some dill around in roasted potatoes or in a salad. It's very low in calories and high in Vitamin C, so feel free to use as much as you want in a dish!

Additional Tips for Growing and Maintaining Dill

If your herb starts to turn yellow, it might mean that it is getting too much water. Keep checking on the water levels inside the soil, and stop watering if it seems like there is too much.

If you don't like the dill flowers or seeds, keep trimming off any flower stalks with clean garden scissors to promote leaf growth.

A blooming plant also takes up a lot of space in your garden, so you will need to keep trimming to ensure it stays in its place.

Lavender

Lavender is one of the most fragrant herbs that you can grow in your garden. It's known for promoting relaxation and helping with sleep.

Light and Water Requirements

Lavender grows really fast when given access to proper sunlight. It also likes water just as much and needs to be watered every day. Keep the soil moist, and water often to ensure the soil does not harden. The summer sun can get too hot sometimes and cause the soil to dry out, making the lavender seem a little droopy. Don't worry, though; just add some mulch and keep maintaining the moisture in your soil to revive it!

The Best Ways to Use Lavender

One thing that pops into your head when someone says lavender is a warm cup of tea!

Baking with lavender is especially common. Here are a few ideas for sweet treats that feature lavender as a major ingredient.

- lavender and honey cookies
- chocolate lavender cake
- vanilla cupcakes with lavender icing
- lemon, lavender, and mascarpone
- lavender and almond scones
- apple and lavender tarts

There are so many more baked goods you can make taste unique with just a little bit of lavender. Get creative by mixing different flavors to create your own special lavender treat. Be careful with the quantity you use, though; a little too much can cause your food to smell and taste like soap!

Other ways to incorporate lavender into your daily routine are homemade lavender creams, infused oils, and other cocktails.

Additional Tips for Growing and Maintaining Lavender

For potted lavender, bottom watering is a simple technique that ensures your plant gets enough water without the risk of drowning it. Allow the soil to dry out a little—it doesn't take long—before you water it again.

Take care not to cut into the woody part of the plant, as it can cause damage.

Mint

Mint has a wide variety of uses, especially in food and drink. Mint-flavored rice tastes excellent too! All you need to do is wash your rice and cook it with some chopped mint and salt!

Light and Water Requirements

If you are growing your mint plant indoors, be sure to put it in a place where it gets a lot of sunlight during the day. Another option is to put it in a cool place and add some grow lights to the area. This way, the soil stays cool, and the artificial lighting provides enough sunlight for the plant to grow well.

Don't go too many days between watering. The soil should not dry out or become hard. Make sure it is always kept moist.

The Best Ways to Use Mint

Mint tea, mojitos, and other drinks are great ways to incorporate mint into your diet. The next time you eat a bowl of fruit, top it up with some mint to give it an extra fresh flavor, especially watermelon.

You can add some mint to any gravy, stuffing, or dessert, including the following examples:

- mint chutney with grilled vegetables
- mint pesto sauce for pasta
- chicken wings with mint sauce
- mint-flavored rice
- mint gravy and lamb
- mint ravioli
- salad dressing
- mint muffins
- chocolate mint mousse
- mint strawberry cake
- mint and cucumber salad
- mojitos
- mint tea

Honestly speaking, you can use mint in any dish you want to make, and it will taste fresh and light and give you an energy boost.

Additional Tips for Growing and Maintaining Mint

Mint tends to overgrow by a lot and occupy as much space as it can get access to. If you are growing your mind along with other plants, be sure it has a confined area or container to prevent it from occupying other plants' spaces.

Oregano

Oregano is native to the Mediterranean region, which is why you'll find it used in a lot of dishes in that cuisine. It is generally an outdoor plant and needs a lot of sunlight to grow well.

Light and Water Requirements

Place your oregano plant in a place with direct access to sunlight. It needs to get at least a couple of hours of sunlight each day. If you are growing it indoors, try to put it close to the window, in an east-facing corner if possible.

Allow the soil to dry out before you water your oregano again. Unlike the other herbs, oregano does not prefer moist soil; it should be a little on the drier side. If it's not a really hot season, watering the plant once a week should be enough. Always check the soil before you water again since it cannot survive when over watered.

The Best Ways to Use Oregano

Oregano is another kind of plant that likes to overgrow, especially when you trim it often. Making fresh organic pesto is a great way to use all the extra herbs that you have left over. It also lasts for quite a few days in the refrigerator and longer in the freezer, so you batch cook a large amount to have delicious pesto all year. Combine your oregano pesto with other flavors like mint, lemon balm, coriander, and others for unique combinations.

You can also top your pizza or tomato sauce with some fresh oregano instead of dried one to give it a better taste.

Herb butter can be made with oregano as well. Just combine some salted butter with finely chopped oregano to give your bread a unique flavor.

Additional Tips for Growing and Maintaining Oregano

Oregano is a natural bug repellent. Place your plant in an area that gets a lot of bugs, especially mosquitoes so it can function as a repellent and protect you.

Parsley

Freshly picked parsley tastes so much better than store-bought or dried parsley. Picking the leaves and immediately using them in your cooking can make a noticeable difference to the flavor and color of your food. It also makes the food much more fragrant.

Light and Water Requirements

Parsley is a very forgiving plant and can survive with less care than other plants. It does well both indoors and outdoors and absorbs both full sun and partial shade.

Water your parsley deeply, at least once a week, or when the soil seems dry to touch. If it is overwatered, you might see it start to turn yellow.

Cut off any yellow stems immediately to allow the plant to grow back well.

It also grows really quickly, so use a bigger pot to make sure the roots grow deep and strong.

The Best Ways to Use Parsley

Parsley works great for any kind of salad. Add some parsley, toss in a few cut veggies, and some chicken for protein, salt, and pepper, and you will have a colorful, fresh salad for a healthy and simple lunch on any day of the week. Here are another few ideas on how to incorporate parsley into your everyday meals.

- parsley-infused rice for your burrito

- lime and parsley chimichurri

- green rice with mint, cilantro, and parsley

- parsley yogurt dip

- avocado and parsley hummus

- tomato soup with parsley

- topping for any stir fry

- gravy

- salmon with a parsley sauce

- ranch dressing

Additional Tips for Growing and Maintaining Parsley

1.   Sowing parsley seeds directly into the soil is the best way to grow them.

2.   Cut the stems an inch away from the soil to help them regrow.

3.   Stop watering if you see it yellowing and check the soil. Move it to a sunny spot to revive it.

4.   Always snip the whole stem instead of just the leaves.

Rosemary

Rosemary takes a little bit of patience if you are trying to grow it from seed. The germination stage can take up to a month or more, depending on the conditions. After repotting, it can take a few more weeks or months before it is ready to be harvested. But its many uses make it definitely worth the effort and wait.

Light and Water Requirements

Rosemary is yet another herb that needs full sunlight. Plant it away from large plants or trees to ensure the roots get enough sunlight in the morning. If there is a lot of shade in your area, the rosemary stems will turn out weak, and the woody part won't taste as great. Try to place your plant in an area that gets a lot of morning sun, since the heat of the afternoon can cause the plant to wilt.

Allow the soil to dry before you water the plant again. This may require you to water it deeply once every few days.

The Best Ways to Use Rosemary

Rosemary has a lot of uses, not just in cooking food but also in its medicinal properties. It is proven (Therapeutic effects of rosemary [*Rosmarinus officinalis* L] and its active constituents on nervous system disorders, 2020) to reduce certain symptoms like nausea, headache, stomachache, and fatigue.

It can be used in a variety of soups, stews, and curries, and it can also be eaten raw in a salad. Pan-sear some rosemary with meats like pork, lamb, or duck breast to give the dish an extra special flavor.

Additional Tips for Growing and Maintaining Rosemary

1. Water rosemary frequently when it is still young and decrease watering as it grows.

2. When planting indoors, place this herb in a humid area.

3. Don't let the soil dry out too much or allow it to get too wet.

Sage

Sage is an herb widely known for its use as a traditional medicine. Some people even find sage to be helpful in cleansing their space and removing bad "aura." It is also widely used in medicine for its antioxidant properties (Hamidpour et al., 2014).

Light and Water Requirements

Sage is low maintenance, grows well in both medium and full sun, and can also grow well in partial shade. It also tolerates drought or desert-like conditions, so you do not need to water it as much as you would water other herbs. Once a week, check the soil to make sure it is not too dry. If it is, add some more water; otherwise, you can go a few more days without watering it. Thoroughly water the plant until you are sure the water has reached the roots and leave it again for another week.

The Best Ways to Use Sage

Sage is a highly fragrant herb and gives off a strong flavor to your dish, even if you add it in the smallest amount. It makes a perfect garnish for any kind of salad or enhances the flavor of a simple soup or stew.

While boiling your pasta, add in some salt and a few leaves of sage to give it an enhanced flavor. Do the same while cooking your sausage: once you remove the casing, cut it up a little, and fry it with sage, salt, and pepper. This can then be used as stuffing for your roast chicken or duck to create a slightly piney and peppery taste.

You can also make quite a few desserts with sage, including

- sage cakes

- sage pie

- panna cotta

- brownies

If you know the right way to use it and are able to estimate a proper quantity, sage can be used almost anywhere!

Additional Tips for Growing and Maintaining Sage

Although sage does survive well under medium sun and partial shade, giving it long hours of sun can make the leaves more flavorful and fresh.

Thyme

Thyme is considered a medicinal herb and has been used since ancient times to cure malaria (Dell'Agli et al., 2012). It is also a well-known herb and is used extensively in British and Italian cuisine.

Light and Water Requirements

Just like sage, thyme also survives on minimal watering, in fact, it likes less watering! A deep watering once every 10 to 15 days should be enough for most areas in the spring and summer. When the summer gets too hot, though, you might need to water the thyme once every 8 to 10 days.

The Best Ways to Use Thyme

There isn't just one way to use thyme; its uses in the culinary world are endless. Most kinds of foods from all around the world—roasts, pan-seared meats, braised vegetables, soups, pastas, cakes—find different uses for thyme.

To cool off in the summer, make yourself a glass of thyme lemonade; it would also make a unique selling point for your kids' lemonade stand! If you like homemade cookies and crackers, thyme fits right into any salted cracker recipe!

Here are a few other dishes where you can add thyme to give them a slight peppery and sweet taste:

- raspberry-thyme jam

- short ribs

- garnish for roasted potatoes

- lemon and thyme roast chicken

- pea puree

- lemon thyme roast salmon

Additional Tips for Growing and Maintaining Thyme

When the plants start to flower, start cutting the flowers off. Leaving the flowers on can slow the growth of the plant and cause it to become woody.

Once you cut off the flower, don't throw it away; instead, clean, dry, and save it. The thyme flower can also be used to make a refreshing tea, which can come in handy when you are looking for natural home remedies to reduce a cold.

Conclusion

Now that you have all the information you need to start your garden, it is time to actually get your hands dirty and start some planting work! As we read in the earlier chapters, it's always important to have a plan for your garden—where you will put your plants, exactly what you want to grow, etc.

After the planning stage comes the most fun part—shopping! This is where you will gather all the material you need to grow and maintain your garden. If you are a beginner, you definitely need a lot of equipment, like pots, soil, seeds, and gardening scissors.

Making a list of everything you need beforehand is a good idea and can save you multiple trips to and from the store. As discussed before, choose the right soil for your plants. Most garden soils, or sandy soils, work best for herb gardens since they do not absorb more water than needed.

If you, for any reason at all, think your soil is not of good quality or are not happy with it, consider making homemade compost to provide some extra nourishment to your soil. Remember, homemade compost takes quite some time and work, so consider getting pre-made compost from the store if you are already well into spring by the time you plan your garden. If you have the time, though, homemade compost is much healthier for your herbs.

It's also a good idea to understand how high your herbs will grow to be able to pick the right-sized pot. Cilantro, for example, might not need that deep of a pot to grow well, but it needs more horizontal space. The mint's roots tend to grow deep, and the plant is large in general. But a very large pot is needed for this herb, since it will take up as much space as you give it.

Germination will be the first thing you do after you come home from buying your plants. If you had a germination tray on your list and bought it, it would make the process of seeding and sprouting much faster and simpler. It's always okay to sow directly into your pot; just make sure you maintain the right temperature and moisture inside the soil for the seed to germinate. If you directly bought a plant, that skips most of the slow steps. All you need to do is repot the plant with your fresh soil and compost mixture.

For germinated plants, once you see them sprout and grow a few centimeters tall, you can transfer them to their new home. Refer to the chapters again if you need to, since this is a crucial step that requires a lot of care. After transferring your plant, secure it tightly in the new soil and water it a little. It takes time for it to adjust, so give the plant all the care you can during this time. Once you pass this step, it's just a few months until you can start using your fresh herbs!

There is one last point that you can't forget, though: the light and water requirements. Be sure to follow all the instructions mentioned in the book to provide your plant with the exact amounts of each that it needs to stay strong and healthy.

In a couple of months, or even less, your herb garden will be fresh and ready for the harvest season! Each plant has its own instructions for harvesting; some need to be harvested close to the root, while others need to be picked at the leaf. To make sure your garden keeps growing, trim it properly, and you always have fresh herbs waiting for you.

During the winter, perennial plants need an extra layer of protection to help them survive the cold. At the end of the day, all living beings are similar. Humans have jackets, animals have fur, and plants need an artificial heat-provider layer. Mulching is a technique of warming plants up during the winter to protect them from frost.

Feel free to refer to this book as many times as you need to, in case you have some questions or doubts about your herbs. For as long as you care for a plant, it will care for you and provide you with food—in this case, flavorful food! Even the simplest of dinners, frozen meals included, can taste restaurant-style when you just toss in a few herbs while heating them up.

Although growing herbs might seem challenging at first, once you get started and figure it all out, it will be one of the most fun and relaxing things that you have ever done! So don't be afraid to take that first step to becoming a gardener; you will thank yourself later! Keep challenging yourself and push yourself to grow more varieties each year.

If you do some research, there are quite a few exotic herbs that you can grow in your garden. Some herbs are simple, like basil and thyme, but some others are quite challenging to maintain. Don't let this scare you, though; there is no reason challenges can't be fun!

For saffron, for example, you need a very large pot and a lot of maintenance to be able to produce less than one gram of saffron, which explains why it's so expensive! If you're up for the challenge, try growing it at home. It can be a new and fun experience overall.

It's always okay if you don't get planting and harvesting right on the first try. What's important is that you keep trying. Remember, gardening is an art; it's one of those good addictions social media talks about! It's not always simple. It's kind of like raising a baby or toddler. The question now is, are you ready to be a plant parent and try a new flavor of food each day?

References

About chive uses, pairings, and recipes. (2023, November 8). *McCormick*. https://www.mccormick.com/articles/mccormick/about-chives#:~:text=Chives%20are%20great%20when%20sprinkled ,fish%2C%20roasted%20chicken%20and%20vegetables

Ajmera, R. (2023, April 6). *10 healthy herbal teas you should try*. Healthline. https://www.healthline.com/nutrition/10-herbal-teas#TOC_TITLE_HDR_10

Akers, C. (2023, May 22). *What is urban gardening?* Earthed. https://www.earthed.co/blog/urban-gardening-is-the-practice-of-growing-plants-fruits-and-vegetables-in-urban-areas/

Alderson, E. (2020, January 9). *How to make herb oil | Naturally Ella*. Naturally Ella. https://naturallyella.com/how-to-make-herb-oil/

Biggs, C. (2021, April 13). How to propagate your favorite herbs, such as rosemary, mint, basil, and more. *Martha Stewart*. https://www.marthastewart.com/8090164/how-propagate-herbs

Bug-Off! Recipes for 4 homemade bug repellents for your skin. (2024, March 14). Almanac.com. https://www.almanac.com/homemade-bug-sprays-stay-bite-free

Burgard, D. (2023, March 14). *When not to prune*. FineGardening. https://www.finegardening.com/project-guides/pruning/when-not-to-prune#:~:text=During%20excessively%20cold%20temperatures&text=It's%20minor%2C%20but%20it%20could,heading%20outside%20to%20the%20garden.

Cahn, L. (2024, February 15). 39 ways to use up that big bunch of parsley. *Taste of Home*. https://www.tasteofhome.com/collection/ways-to-use-up-parsley/

Challenge Dairy. (2023, November 28). *Fresh herb gravy*. *Challenge Dairy*. https://challengedairy.com/recipes/side-dishes/fresh-herb-gravy/

Chappell, S. (2019, December 18). *A beginner's guide to making herbal salves and lotions*. Healthline. https://www.healthline.com/health/diy-herbal-salves#TOC_TITLE_HDR_1

Comfort Keepers. (n.d.). *Herbal gardening and its benefits | Comfort keepers*. https://www.comfortkeepers.com/articles/info-center/senior-independent-living/herbal-gardening-and-its-benefits/

Covington, L. (2024, March 20). *How to dry herbs: 4 simple ways*. The Spruce Eats. https://www.thespruceeats.com/harvesting-and-drying-leafy-herbs-1327541

Currie, J. (2024, March 22). The 12 Best Grow Lights of 2024, Tested and Reviewed. *The Spruce*. https://www.thespruce.com/best-grow-lights-4158720

Defining sun requirements for plants. (n.d.). https://www.johnson.k-state.edu/lawn-garden/agent-articles/miscellaneous/defining-sun-requirements-for-plants.html

Dell'Agli, M., Sanna, C., Rubiolo, P., Basilico, N., Colombo, E., Scaltrito, M., Ndiath, M. O., Maccarone, L., Taramelli, D., Bicchi, C., Ballero, M., & Bosisio, E. (2012). Anti-plasmodial and insecticidal activities of the essential oils of aromatic plants growing in the Mediterranean area. *Malaria Journal, 11*(1). https://doi.org/10.1186/1475-2875-11-219

Department of Health & Human Services. (n.d.). *Herbs.* Better Health Channel.
https://www.betterhealth.vic.gov.au/health/healthyliving/herbs

Ellen. (2012, April 19). *Herb Flavour Chart.* Eat Well. https://canolaeatwell.com/herb-flavour-chart/

Food & Wine Editors. (2022, September 8). 21 Recipes for mint Lovers. *Food & Wine.* https://www.foodandwine.com/seasonings/herbs/mint/mint

Foster, K. (2022, March 14). *20+ delicious ways to use up a bunch of parsley.* Kitchn. https://www.thekitchn.com/parsley-recipes-246217

4 ways to dry your homegrown tea herbs + how to store them properly! (n.d.). DIY Herbal Tea. https://www.diyherbaltea.com/how-to-dry-herbs.html

Fung, T. K., Lau, B. W., Ngai, S. P., & Tsang, H. W. H. (2021). Therapeutic Effect and Mechanisms of Essential Oils in Mood Disorders: Interaction between the Nervous and Respiratory Systems. *International Journal of Molecular Sciences, 22*(9), 4844. https://doi.org/10.3390/ijms22094844

Gardening Statistics (2024). (2022, September 5). RubyHome.com. https://www.rubyhome.com/blog/gardening-stats/

GeeksforGeeks. (2024, March 19). *Top 10 largest spice producing countries in the world.* GeeksforGeeks. https://www.geeksforgeeks.org/largest-spice-producing-countries-in-the-world/

Gordon Ramsay. (2018, December 10). *Roast a turkey with Gordon Ramsay* [Video]. YouTube. https://www.youtube.com/watch?v=XO5DF8soxwM

Greendigs. (n.d.). *Your guide to: Oregano.* https://shopgreendigs.com/plant-care/your-guide-to-oregano.html

Gregarious Inc. (2022a, January 22). *Italian parsley plant care: water, light, nutrients | Greg App* . Greg App 🌱. https://greg.app/plant-care/italian-parsely#fertilizer-repotting-needs

Gregarious Inc. (2022b, March 9). *Lavender care 101: water, light & growing tips.* Greg App 🌱. https://greg.app/plant-care/lavandula-stoechas-lavender

Growing chives. (2011, October 2). Bonnie Plants. https://bonnieplants.com/blogs/how-to-grow/growing-chives

Growing chives in home gardens. (n.d.-a). UMN Extension. https://extension.umn.edu/vegetables/growing-chives#harvesting-934461

Growing chives in home gardens. (n.d.-b). UMN Extension. https://extension.umn.edu/vegetables/growing-chives#:~:text=testing%20and%20fertilizer-,Chives%20thrive%20in%20full%20sun%20and%20well%20drained%20soil%20rich,of%20direct%20light%20is%20best

Growing parsley in home gardens. (n.d.). UMN Extension. https://extension.umn.edu/vegetables/growing-parsley

A guide to common medicinal herbs. (Anon) *Health Encyclopedia,* University of Rochester Medical Center. (n.d.). https://www.urmc.rochester.edu/encyclopedia/content.aspx?contenttypeid=1&contentid=1169

A guide to watering herbs—best practices for a healthy herb garden. (2022, March 24). Swan Hose. https://swanhose.com/blogs/watering-herbs/a-guide-to-watering-herbs-best-practices-for-a-healthy-herb-garden

Hamidpour, M., Hamidpour, R., Hamidpour, S., & Shahlari, M. (2014). Chemistry, pharmacology, and medicinal property of sage (salvia) to prevent and cure illnesses such as obesity, diabetes, depression, dementia, lupus, autism, heart disease, and cancer. *Journal of Traditional and Complementary Medicine, 4*(2), 82–88.

https://doi.org/10.4103/2225-4110.130373

Hardening off tender plants / RHS Gardening. (n.d.). Royal Horticultural Society. https://www.rhs.org.uk/prevention-protection/hardening-off-tender-plants

Hardening off vegetable seedlings for the home garden. (n.d.). University of Maryland Extension. https://extension.umd.edu/resource/hardening-vegetable-seedlings-home-garden/

Harvard Health. (2021, October 21). *The health benefits of 3 herbal teas.* https://www.health.harvard.edu/nutrition/the-health-benefits-of-3-herbal-teas

Hassani, N. (2024, April 8). *How to water plants: 20 essential tips.* The Spruce. https://www.thespruce.com/tips-for-watering-plants-5198467

Health benefits of basil. (2023, July 2). WebMD. https://www.webmd.com/diet/health-benefits-basil

Health benefits of mint leaves. (2023, February 14). WebMD. https://www.webmd.com/diet/health-benefits-mint-leaves

Health benefits of parsley. (2022, November 27). WebMD. https://www.webmd.com/diet/health-benefits-parsley

Herbal medicine. (n.d.). Mount Sinai Health System. https://www.mountsinai.org/health-library/treatment/herbal-

medicine#:~:text=What%20is%20herbal%20medicine%20goo
d,%2C%20and%20cancer%2C%20among%20others

Hirneisen, A., & LaBorde, L. (n.d.). *Let's preserve: drying herbs.* PennState
Extension. Retrieved July 31, 2023, from
https://extension.psu.edu/lets-preserve-drying-herbs

Hirneisen, A., MA. (n.d.). *Let's preserve drying herbs.*
https://extension.psu.edu/lets-preserve-drying-
herbs#:~:text=Preparing%20Herbs%20for%20Drying&text=
Remove%20any%20bruised%2C%20soiled%2C%20or,dry%20
with%20a%20paper%20towel.

Holy basil tea: Are there health benefits? (2022, September 8). WebMD.
https://www.webmd.com/diet/holy-basil-tea-health-benefits

How to choose what soil is right for your garden. (n.d.).
https://anlscape.com.au/.
https://anlscape.com.au/advice/gardening/how-to-choose-
what-soil-is-right-for-your-
garden#:~:text=Generally%20soils%20should%20be%20well,
have%20an%20earthy%20moist%20smell

How to grow basil plants: The complete guide. (2024, March 27). Almanac.com.
https://www.almanac.com/plant/basil

How to keep herb plants fresh, beautiful and well hydrated | Chrysal. (n.d.).
https://www.chrysal.com/tips/tips/how-keep-herb-plants-
fresh-beautiful-and-well-
hydrated#:~:text=Put%20your%20herb%20plant%20in,sure%
20it%20has%20enough%20water

How to water your plants. (n.d.). https://www.longfield-gardens.com/article/how-to-water-your-plants

How urban gardens create greener, healthier cities. (n.d.). The Wilderness Society. https://www.wilderness.org/articles/blog/how-urban-gardens-create-greener-healthier-cities

Huggins, R. (2020, March 12). *Fresh herb marinade* -. https://thecampgroundgourmet.com/fresh-herb-marinade/

Iorfino, R. (2023, November 10). *The best herb garden design for your backyard.* Better Homes and Gardens. https://www.bhg.com.au/layout-herb-garden-design

Juddlefeber. (2020, October 23). *What if you don't have enough sun? – Green thumb gardening Secrets.* https://greenthumbgardeningsecrets.com/what-if-you-dont-have-enough-sun/

June, C. (2021, November 27). How to cook with lavender so your food doesn't taste like soap. *Bon Appétit.* https://www.bonappetit.com/test-kitchen/how-to/article/cooking-with-lavender

Jusek, J. (2022, January 5). 30 Recipes You Can Make with Fresh Thyme. *Taste of Home.* https://www.tasteofhome.com/collection/recipes-with-fresh-thyme/

Kate. (2020, March 30). *How to make vinaigrette (Plus 3 essential variations!).* Cookie and Kate. https://cookieandkate.com/how-to-make-vinaigrette-plus-variations/

Kyla. (2024, March 12). *Rosemary oil for hair growth: Benefits + how to make it 3 ways.* A Life Adjacent. https://alifeadjacent.com/rosemary-oil-for-hair-growth/

Lambton, C. (2022, April 4). *The ultimate guide to growing, caring for & harvesting basil plants.* https://www.fiskars.com/en-us/gardening-and-yard-care/ideas-and-how-tos/planting-and-prep/growing-basil-planting-and-harvesting#:~:text=Basil%20prefers%20moist%20soil%20%E2%80%93%20not,shade%20over%20your%20basil%20plant

Laura. (2022, June 29). *Fresh herb salsa verde.* A Beautiful Plate. https://www.abeautifulplate.com/fresh-herb-salsa-verde/

Lindblad, A. J., & Koppula, S. (2016, February 1). *Ginger for nausea and vomiting of pregnancy.* PubMed Central (PMC). https://www.ncbi.nlm.nih.gov/pmc/articles/PMC4755634/

Lipford, D. (2024, February 2). *Annual and perennial herbs for your garden.* Today's Homeowner. https://todayshomeowner.com/lawn-garden/guides/annual-and-perennial-herbs-for-your-garden/

Littlewood, N. (2024a, February 20). *How to grow herbs from seed successfully every time.* Urban Leaf. https://www.geturbanleaf.com/blogs/care/how-to-grow-herbs-from-seeds#:~:text=If%20you%20are%20starting%20to,some%20sort%20of%20germination%20tray.&text=Although%20these%20are%20available%20as,covers%20a%20few%20such%20ideas

Littlewood, N. (2024b, February 20). *How to grow herbs from seed successfully every time.* Urban Leaf. https://www.geturbanleaf.com/blogs/care/how-to-grow-herbs-from-seeds#:~:text=If%20you%20are%20starting%20to,some%20sort%20of%20germination%20tray.&text=Although%20these%20are%20available%20as,covers%20a%20few%20such%20ideas

Lotfi, A., Mohtashami, J., Khangholi, Z. A., & Shirmohammadi-Khorram, N. (2020). The efficacy of aromatherapy with lemon balm (Melissa officinalis L.) on sleep quality in cardiac patients: a randomized controlled trial. *Research Square (Research Square).* https://doi.org/10.21203/rs.3.rs-68416/v1

MacArthur, A. (2024, March 28). *How to make homemade fertilizer for indoor herbs.* Food Gardening Network. https://foodgardening.mequoda.com/daily/soil-fertilizer/how-to-make-homemade-fertilizer-for-indoor-herbs/#:~:text=Making%20homemade%20fertilizer%20for%20indoor%20herbs%20in%20the%20kitchen&text=Boiling%20potatoes%20and%20other%20vegetables,the%20soil%20around%20your%20herbs

Mair, C. (n.d.). City life: Why are green spaces important? Natural HistoryMuseum.https://www.nhm.ac.uk/discover/why-we-need-green-spaces-in-cities.html#:~:text=Green%20spaces%20in%20cities%20mitig ate,a%20result%20of%20human%20activity

Make your own herb butter to add flavor to almost anything. (2024, February 22). The Spruce Eats. https://www.thespruceeats.com/herb-butter-recipe-1327883

MasterClass. (2021, August 13). *How to cook with sage: 11 culinary uses for sage - 2024 - MasterClass.* https://www.masterclass.com/articles/how-to-cook-with-sage-11-culinary-uses-for-sage

MasterClass. (2022, September 2). *Cooking 101: The 15 most common culinary herbs and how to cook with them - 2024 - MasterClass.* https://www.masterclass.com/articles/cooking-101-the-15-most-common-culinary-herbs-and-how-to-cook-with-them

McCann, D. (2021, June 8). How to trim your herbs and why you need to. *Allrecipes.* https://www.allrecipes.com/article/how-to-trim-herbs/

McGrane, K. (2020, February 4). *All you need to know about dill.* Healthline. https://www.healthline.com/nutrition/dill#uses

Mike. (2016, June 8). *65 Inspiring DIY herb gardens - Shelterness.* Shelterness. https://www.shelterness.com/40-inspiring-diy-herb-gardens/

Mittal, N. (2023, July 17). *Tea culture in Germany.* Mittal Teas. https://mittalteas.com/blogs/news/tea-culture-in-germany#:~:text=Herbal%20Tea%20Tradition%3A%20Germany%20has,for%20their%20perceived%20health%20benefits.

Monkeys and medicinal plants. (2014, October 21). Nature. https://www.pbs.org/wnet/nature/clever-monkeys-monkeys-and-medicinal-plants/3957/

Overwatered vs underwatered plants: signs, fix tips (Full Guide). (n.d.). PlantIn. https://myplantin.com/blog/overwatered-vs-underwatered-plants

Pagán, C. N. (2024, April 6). *What is aromatherapy?* WebMD. https://www.webmd.com/balance/stress-management/aromatherapy-overview

Pangborn, L. (2023, July 18). *5 telltale signs of overwatered plants, according to the grow-how team.* Bloomscape. https://bloomscape.com/plant-care/telltale-signs-of-overwatered-plants-according-to-plant-mom/#:~:text=If%20a%20plant%20is%20overwatered,sign%20of%20too%20little%20water)

PEPPERMINT: Overview, uses, side effects, precautions, interactions, dosing and reviews. (n.d.). https://www.webmd.com/vitamins/ai/ingredientmono-705/peppermint

Prepare your plants for winter. (n.d.). News. https://www.extension.iastate.edu/news/2009/oct/061201.htm

Preserving herbs by freezing or drying. (n.d.). UMN Extension. https://extension.umn.edu/preserving-and-preparing/preserving-herbs-freezing-or-drying#:~:text=Store%20in%20airtight%20containers,-Place%20them%20in&text=Glass%20keeps%20aromas%20in.,year%20in%20refrigerators%20or%20freezers.

Professional, C. C. M. (n.d.). *Aromatherapy*. Cleveland Clinic. https://my.clevelandclinic.org/health/treatments/aromatherapy

Rada, R. (2018, July 5). *Herbs sunlight chart: 15 most popular herbs and their sunlight requirements*. The Happy Gardening Life. https://thehappygardeninglife.com/blogs/organic-gardening/herbs-sunlight-chart

Rahbardar, M. G., & Hosseinzadeh, H. (2020). Therapeutic effects of rosemary (Rosmarinus officinalis L.) and its active constituents on nervous system disorders. *PubMed*, *23*(9), 1100–1112. https://doi.org/10.22038/ijbms.2020.45269.10541

Raman, R. (2024, April 9). *12 health benefits and uses of sage*. Healthline. https://www.healthline.com/nutrition/sage#:~:text=Sage%20is%20an%20herb%20with,dried%20or%20as%20a%20tea

Rankel, K. (2023, December 16). *Light requirements for your dill*. Greg App. https://greg.app/dill-light-requirements/#:~:text=Full%20sun%20is%20key%3A%20Dill,shade%20to%20mimic%20shorter%20days

Rhoades, H. (2021, June 23). *Watering rosemary for rosemary plant care.* Gardeningknowhow. https://www.gardeningknowhow.com/edible/herbs/rosemary /watering-rosemary.htm

Roselli, E. (2023, July 11). *How to trim your herbs and keep them happy!* Hicks Nurseries. https://hicksnurseries.com/herbs-and-vegetables/how-to-trim-your-herbs-and-keep-them-happy/#:~:text=Snip%20leaves%20from%20annual%20herbs, an%20inch%20from%20the%20soil.

Rothenberg, D. O., & Zhang, L. (2019). Mechanisms underlying the Anti-Depressive effects of regular tea consumption. *Nutrients, 11*(6), 1361. https://doi.org/10.3390/nu11061361

Roxburgh, L. (2024, February 14). *Best herbal cocktails to try.* Good Food. https://www.bbcgoodfood.com/howto/guide/best-herbal-cocktails-to-try

Russell, P. (2018, September 9). *How to dry herbs.* Instructables. https://www.instructables.com/How-to-Dry-Herbs/

Sánchez, E., PhD. (n.d.). *Herb and spice history.* https://extension.psu.edu/herb-and-spice-history#:~:text=The%20United%20States%20produces%20ab out,herbs%20and%20spices%20per%20year.

Schill, J. (2021, October 26). How to Protect Plants from Frost: Coverage That Works. *Green Inpressions.* https://www.mygreenimpressions.com/blog/bid/321963/how -to-cover-plants-for-frost-protection

seedling.   (2024).
https://dictionary.cambridge.org/dictionary/english/seedling

Should you mulch in the winter. (2024, April 4). Gecko Green Lawn Care & Pest Control. https://geckogreen.com/should-you-mulch-in-the-winter#:~:text=Choosing%20the%20Right%20Mulch%20for, benefits%20in%20enhancing%20soil%20fertility.

Should you use a Self-Watering pot? (2022, July 18). Living Color Garden Center. https://livingcolorgardencenter.net/gardening/using-self-watering-pots/#:~:text=Plenty%20of%20plants%20can%20do,the%20 bottom%2Dup%20watering%20system

Sill. (n.d.). *How often & how much you should water houseplants.* The Sill. https://www.thesill.com/blog/drink-up

Spice, P. (2023, February 2). *Fascinating facts about 10 herbs and spices - PSC.* Pacific Spice Company. https://pacificspice.com/2023/01/25/fascinating-facts-about-10-herbs-spices/

Staff, S. L. P. (2023, October 24). Southern living plants. *Southern Living Plants.* https://southernlivingplants.com/planting-care/when-to-water/#:~:text=Morning%20watering%20is%20actually%20pr eferable,%2C%20fungal%20growth%2C%20and%20insects.

Stevinson, C., Pittler, M. H., & Ernst, E. (2000). Garlic for treating hypercholesterolemia. *Annals of Internal Medicine, 133*(6), 420.

https://doi.org/10.7326/0003-4819-133-6-200009190-00009

Studioplant.com. (n.d.). *How much sunlight does a indoor plant need?* https://www.studioplant.com/de_en/blog/how-much-sunlight-does-a-indoor-plant-need#:~:text=Too%20much%20light%20will%20burn,often%20hang%20down%20a%20bit.

Svedi, R. (2021, June 10). *The top ten benefits of growing your own herb garden.* Gardeningknowhow. https://www.gardeningknowhow.com/edible/herbs/hgen/the-top-ten-benefits-of-growing-your-own-herb-garden.htm

10 best lavender Baking Recipes | Yummly. (n.d.). Yummly. https://www.yummly.com/recipes/lavender-baking10 golden rules for watering. (n.d.). https://www.gardena.com/int/c/discover/gardening/magazine/10-golden-rules-for-watering

The brief history of container gardening. blog. (n.d.). https://www.kawvalleygreenhouses.com/blog/Detail/the-brief-history-of-container-gardening#:~:text=Gardening%20dates%20all%20the%20way,signified%20the%20beginning%20of%20civilization

The ultimate guide to growing herbs. Gardenary. (n.d.). https://www.gardenary.com/blog/the-ultimate-guide-to-growing-herbs

THYME: Overview, uses, side effects, precautions, interactions, dosing and reviews. (n.d.). https://www.webmd.com/vitamins/ai/ingredientmono-

823/thyme

Tips on Cooking with Fresh Herbs. (n.d.). University of Maryland Extension. https://extension.umd.edu/resource/tips-cooking-fresh-herbs/

Todd, L. (2021, June 30). *10 of the healthiest herbs and spices and their health benefits.* https://www.medicalnewstoday.com/articles/healthy-herbs-and-spices#peppermint

Thompson, R. (2018). Gardening for health: a regular dose of gardening. *Clinical Medicine,* *18*(3), 201–205. https://doi.org/10.7861/clinmedicine.18-3-201

Tonia. (2021, January 25). *Make your own herbal tea blends!* Feasting at Home. https://www.feastingathome.com/herbal-tea-recipes/

Trudy. (2017, November 8). *Gardening as exercise.* MPCP. https://www.mpcp.com/articles/healthy-lifestyle/gardening-as-exercise/#:~:text=Yes%2C%20indeed.,build%20strength%20and%20burn%20calories

12 Health benefits of thyme. (2023, May 30). Healthline. https://www.healthline.com/health/health-benefits-of-thyme

2024 Frost dates: First and last frost dates by ZIP code | The Old Farmer's Almanac. (n.d.). Almanac.com. https://www.almanac.com/gardening/frostdates

Uronnachi, E., Atuegwu, C., Umeyor, C., Nwakile, C., Obasi, J., Ikeotuonye, C., & Attama, A. A. (2022a). Formulation and evaluation of hair growth enhancing effects of oleogels made from Rosemary and Cedar wood oils. *Scientific African, 16,* e01223. https://doi.org/10.1016/j.sciaf.2022.e01223

Uronnachi, E., Atuegwu, C., Umeyor, C., Nwakile, C., Obasi, J., Ikeotuonye, C., & Attama, A. A. (2022b). Formulation and evaluation of hair growth enhancing effects of oleogels made from rosemary and cedarwood oils. *Scientific African, 16,* e01223. https://doi.org/10.1016/j.sciaf.2022.e01223

Verena. (2023, June 22). *Herbs that grow in full sun: 13 sun-loving herbs - Plantura.* Plantura. https://plantura.garden/uk/herbs/growing-herbs/herbs-that-grow-in-full-sun

Vertical herb gardens. (n.d.). Pinterest. https://www.pinterest.com/balconygardenwe/vertical-herb-gardens/

Weaver, C. (2023, April 24). Gentle methods for the hard work of gardening. *Voice of America.* https://learningenglish.voanews.com/a/gentle-methods-for-the-hard-work-of-gardening/7057249.html

What is mulching? (2017, April 30). *J K Cooper Tree Services.* https://www.jkcooper.com.au/what-is-mulching/#:~:text=Mulching%20is%20a%20widely%2Dpracticed,the%20condition%20of%20the%20soil.

Wilkes, L. A. (2023, April 19). *Herb pasta (30 minute meal)*. Your Homebased Mom. https://www.yourhomebasedmom.com/herbed-pasta/

Wimmer, L. (2022, July 12). *Dig into the benefits of gardening*. Mayo Clinic Health System. https://www.mayoclinichealthsystem.org/hometown-health/speaking-of-health/dig-into-the-benefits-of-gardening

Made in the USA
Las Vegas, NV
26 July 2024